Public Health in the 21st Century

Neglected Tropical Diseases: Background, Identification and Prevention

PUBLIC HEALTH IN THE 21ST CENTURY

Additional books in this series can be found on Nova's website under the Series tab.

Additional E-books in this series can be found on Nova's website under the E-books tab.

PUBLIC HEALTH IN THE 21ST CENTURY

NEGLECTED TROPICAL DISEASES: BACKGROUND, IDENTIFICATION AND PREVENTION

RONALD J. DAVIDSON

EDITOR

Nova Science Publishers, Inc.
New York

For permission to use material from this book please contact us:
Telephone 631-231-7269; Fax 631-231-8175
Web Site: http://www.novapublishers.com

NOTICE TO THE READER

Library of Congress Cataloging-in-Publication Data

Neglected tropical diseases : background, identification and prevention / editor, Ronald J. Davidson.
p. ; cm.
Includes bibliographical references and index.
ISBN 978-1-61324-387-9 (softcover : alk. paper) 1. Tropical medicine. I. Davidson, Ronald J.
[DNLM: 1. Neglected Diseases--prevention & control--Collected Works. 2. Tropical Medicine--Collected Works. 3. Neglected Diseases--diagnosis--Collected Works. WC 680]
RC961.N44 2011
616.9'883--dc22

2011012560

Published by Nova Science Publishers, Inc. ✝ New York

CONTENTS

PREFACE

Over the past decade, global health has become a priority in U.S. foreign policy, and U.S. funding for related efforts has more than tripled. Neglected tropical diseases (NTDs), an important focus of U.S. global health assistance, may come under scrutiny as the 112th Congress debates spending levels for ongoing global health programs. Estimates indicate that some 2 billion people are at risk of contracting an NTD, of whom more than 1 billion people are afflicted with one or more. This book examines the background, responses and issues for Congress relating to Neglected Tropical Diseases (NTDs), while identifying research gaps and opportunities.

Chapter 1- Over the past decade, global health has become a priority in U.S. foreign policy, and U.S. funding for related efforts has more than tripled. Neglected tropical diseases (NTDs), an important focus of U.S. global health assistance, may come under scrutiny as the 112th Congress debates spending levels for ongoing global health programs. NTDs are a group of 17 diseases that are found primarily among the poorest people in 149 countries and territories. Estimates indicate that some 2 billion people are at risk of contracting an NTD, of whom more than 1 billion people are afflicted with one or more. Roughly 534,000 people are believed to be killed by an NTD annually.

Chapter 2- Tropical diseases have been part of the NIH mission since its founding and are incorporated into the Public Health Service Act as part of the NIH mission. International collaborative efforts as well as public-private partnerships are generating new opportunities for making substantial progress in novel interventions for many infectious diseases of the tropics. Growing public interest in global health could add to this momentum. International efforts in malaria, tuberculosis and HIV are providing an infrastructure that overlaps geographically with endemic areas for many other infectious diseases, creating prospects for shared research capabilities and opportunities. The availability of new methodological approaches such as genomics, proteomics, synthetic chemistry, molecular and genetic epidemiology, as well as increases in information and communication technologies, may further enhance prospects for progress in research on many infectious diseases found in the tropics. Although many such diseases have been historically thought of as resulting from poverty, they have been more recently recognized as a significant cause of poverty that must be addressed in order to break the cycle of poverty.

Chapter 3- At present, 884 million people do not have access to improved water sources and 2.6 billion people lack access to improved sanitation.[1] At any given time, close to half the people living in the developing world are suffering from one or more diseases associated with inadequate water, sanitation, and hygiene (WASH).[2] The most recognized WASH disease is diarrheal illness, which causes more than 1.5 million deaths worldwide every year, mostly among children younger than five years of age.[3] Millions more suffer from devastating WASH-related neglected tropical diseases (NTDs), such as soil-transmitted helminthiases (STHs), Guinea worm disease (GWD), trachoma, and schistosomiasis.

In: Neglected Tropical Diseases
Editor: Ronald J. Davidson ISBN: 978-1-61324-387-9

Chapter 1

NEGLECTED TROPICAL DISEASES: BACKGROUND, RESPONSES, AND ISSUES FOR CONGRESS*

Tiaji Salaam-Blyther

SUMMARY

Over the past decade, global health has become a priority in U.S. foreign policy, and U.S. funding for related efforts has more than tripled. Neglected tropical diseases (NTDs), an important focus of U.S. global health assistance, may come under scrutiny as the 112th Congress debates spending levels for ongoing global health programs. NTDs are a group of 17 diseases that are found primarily among the poorest people in 149 countries and territories. Estimates indicate that some 2 billion people are at risk of contracting an NTD, of whom more than 1 billion people are afflicted with one or more. Roughly 534,000 people are believed to be killed by an NTD annually.

Although these diseases are concentrated among the world's poor, population shifts and climate change increase the vulnerability of the United States to some of these diseases, particularly Chagas disease and dengue. While blood centers test for Chagas, some health experts believe that several cases remain undiagnosed in the United States and that Chagas stands as an undetected cause of heart disease and stroke. Some

* This is an edited, reformatted and augmented version of a Congressional Research Services publication, dated January 21, 2011.

observers are concerned about scientists' expectations that mosquitoes capable of spreading dengue fever are gradually spreading across the United States, particularly because no vaccine or treatment exists for this disease. In addition, travelers from industrialized countries are increasingly contracting NTDs such as schistosomiasis while engaged in tourism. These cases are usually identified once tourists develop severe, acute infection or other unusual problems.

Proponents support funding research on and treatment for NTDs because it is a cost-effective way of making a significant health impact. Roughly 90% of all NTDs are easy to treat with drugs that cost less than $2 per dose and need to be taken only once or twice annually. This means that all people at risk of contracting an NTD worldwide can be treated for less than $2 billion over the next five years. With consistent treatment and control, several NTDs are being eliminated in various parts of the world, especially in Latin America, and guinea worm disease is on the cusp of eradication, meaning there is no risk of contracting the disease.

Some groups argue that the United States should increase funding for NTD programs to improve global health and advance domestic capacity to detect NTD cases that may arise, particularly for diseases like dengue and Chagas. Other groups maintain that countries like Brazil, China, and India that have received support for eliminating NTDs should play a greater role in addressing the health challenge, particularly as their own economies exhibit strong growth. The 112th Congress may debate funding much of the President's FY2011 budget, which includes $155 million for the NTD Program, as well as upcoming FY2012 budget levels. The 112th Congress will likely weigh calls for greater spending on NTDs with other challenges, such as streamlining foreign and global health assistance to make them more effective and efficient, particularly in light of efforts to reduce federal spending.

BACKGROUND

Over the past decade, global health has become a priority in U.S. foreign policy, and U.S. appropriations for health-related efforts have more than tripled. Some observers expect the 112th Congress to debate the appropriate funding level for ongoing global health programs, to consider ways to make U.S. global health initiatives more effective and efficient, and to encourage other players to become more engaged, particularly countries such as China and India that are receiving assistance from donors to address health challenges while their economies are undergoing considerable growth.

Neglected tropical diseases (NTDs) have become an important part of U.S. global health assistance, particularly since 2006, when Congress made available $15 million to combat such diseases and President George W. Bush launched the NTD Program. NTDs comprise a group of 17 diseases found mostly among the poorest in 149 countries and territories, primarily in areas with unsafe water, inadequate sanitation, and limited health services. (See *Appendix C* for a description of NTDs, including their symptoms and prevalence; *Appendix D* displays their images). The list is not exhaustive of all illnesses found among this population, but it accounts for those being targeted by the World Health Organization (WHO) and its partners.

Some diseases are transmitted by people; others are spread by vectors like snails, flies, or mosquitoes; and several others are found in contaminated sources (like infested soil or water). [1] At the same time that NTDs afflict primarily the impoverished, some studies indicate that NTDs exacerbate poverty.[2] People crippled by lymphatic filariasis (elephantiasis), for example, often cease to be employable or capable of engaging in income-producing activities. Children afflicted with soil-transmitted helminths (STH) have reduced cognitive functions, poorer health and nutrition, and lower school attendance rates. All of these factors reduce lifetime earning potential.

In 2003, WHO convened a meeting to discuss challenges in addressing a host of tropical diseases that were widely viewed to be receiving inadequate attention and worsening poverty.[3] Though efforts to address these diseases preceded the meeting, up until that point, national governments and global health groups had focused on each of the diseases separately. Following the meeting, WHO and other health experts dubbed a group of 17 infections "neglected tropical diseases" because data showed that people tended to be infected with more than one of these maladies at once. At least 100 countries face two endemic NTD disease burdens, for example, and 30 countries carry six or more NTD endemic disease burdens *(Figure 1).*

Though NTDs are a group of distinct diseases, they share three key characteristics. Specifically, NTDs

- **are long-standing health problems** that have afflicted human beings for centuries, have virtually disappeared in industrialized countries, and have continued to primarily affect the world's poorest populations;
- **cause chronic conditions** that have relatively low mortality rates but may bring long-lasting deformities, which are irreversible in some cases, and impair health, quality of life, and earning potential; and
- **could benefit from greater research and development (R&D).** Additional research could identify second-line treatments that could

be used should the diseases become resistant against drugs. R&D could also identify treatments for incurable ailments like dengue fever and buruli ulcer. For other NTDs like sleeping sickness, innovative research could be used to develop medicines that could supplant commonly used drugs that are toxic, have complex treatment regimens, and carry significant side effects (including death). For all of the NTDs, R&D could be used to identify a vaccine and develop improved diagnostic tools that could be easily used in low-resource settings.

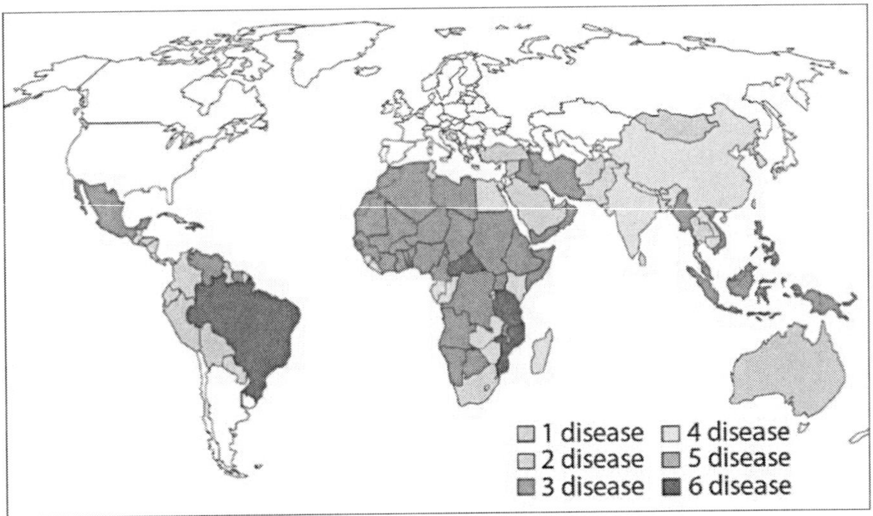

Source: David Molyneux, Peter Hotez, and Alan Fenwick, "Rapid-Impact Interventions": How a Policy of Integrated Control for Africa's Neglected Tropical Diseases Could Benefit the Poor," *PLoS Medicine*, vol. 2, no. 11 (November 2005), pp. 1064-1070.

Figure 1. Global Distribution of NTDs.

Health experts reconvened in 2005 and developed a framework for implementing an integrative approach to controlling NTDs, which focused on three key strategies:

- **Preventive Chemotherapy** through mass drug administration (MDA)—administering treatments to an affected population irrespective of individual disease status.

- **Vector control**—limiting or eradicating disease-carrying insects to reduce transmission of NTDs.
- **Disease surveillance and care**—improving the monitoring of NTD cases and the care of those carrying the diseases.[4]

PREVALENCE

The best available estimates indicate that some 2 billion people are at risk of contracting an NTD, of whom more than 1 billion people are afflicted with one or more NTD. Roughly 534,000 are killed by an NTD annually (*Table 1*).[5]

Despite the common use of the estimates cited above, health experts do not know exactly how many people are infected with NTDs. Uncertainty regarding the number of people suffering from NTDs is rooted in several issues. The majority of people living with NTDs live in marginalized communities that lack sufficient health care, possibly obscuring a diagnosis. The full extent of the global NTD burden may also be hidden behind the symptoms that NTDs cause. Schistosomiasis, for example, can cause anemia and bladder cancer. Additionally, weak health systems may fail to document the true burden of NTDs. One study estimates that one NTD case is reported for every 40 occurrences.[6]

In addition, health information systems in many developing countries are in poor condition and are not equipped to provide precise data on disease prevalence. As such, disease assessments in developing countries, particularly in sub-Saharan Africa, are often based on projections extrapolated from household surveys rather than medical records establishing a diagnosis. Disease prevalence mapping for NTDs has reportedly been improving, however, as the international community boosts investments in addressing NTDs. According to the U.S. Agency for International Development (USAID), by the end of 2009, the NTD burden of the seven most common NTDs had been identified in most districts throughout the countries supported by the United States *(Figure 2)*.

Table 1. Estimated Prevalence of and Deaths Caused by 12 Most Common NTDs

Disease	Prevalence (millions)	Annual Deaths	Most Affected Region
Soil-transmitted helminths			
Ascariasis (roundworm)	807	3,000-60,000	South and East Asia/Pacific, Latin America, and sub-Saharan Africa
Trichuriasis (whipworm)	604	3,000-10,000	South and East Asia/Pacific, Latin America, and sub-Saharan Africa
Hookworm	576	3,000-65,000	South and East Asia/Pacific, Latin America, and sub-Saharan Africa
Schistosomiasis (snail fever)	207	150,000-200,000	Latin America and sub-Saharan Africa
Lymphatic Filariasis (elephantiasis)	120	<500	South and East Asia/Pacific, and sub-Saharan Africa
Dengue/Dengue Fever	50	12,500	Tropical Regions
Trachoma	84	<500	East Asia/Pacific, Latin America, Middle East/North Africa, and sub-Saharan Africa
Onchocerciasis (river blindness)	37	<500	Latin America and sub-Saharan Africa
Leishmaniasis	12	51,000	South Asia, Latin America, and sub-Saharan Africa
Chagas Disease	8.5	14,000	Latin America

Disease	Prevalence (millions)	Annual Deaths	Most Affected Region
Leprosy	0.4	6,000	India, Latin America, and sub-Saharan Africa
Human African Trypanosomiasis (sleeping sickness)	0.3	48,000	Sub-Saharan Africa
Buruli Ulcer	0.05	Unknown	Sub-Saharan Africa
Dracunculiasis (guinea worm)	0.01	Unknown	Sub-Saharan Africa

Source: Peter Hotez, *Forgotten People, Forgotten Diseases* (Washington, DC: ASM Press, 2008), pp. 5, 106, and WHO, *Dengue and Dengue Haemorrhagic Fever*, Fact Sheet 117, March 2009.

Note: These figures should not be aggregated since people are often infected with more than one NTD at once. The three STH are counted as one disease. Five other NTDs are not included here because data on prevalence, morbidity, and mortality are limited. These are rabies, cysticercosis, echinococcosis, endemic treponematoses (yaws), and foodborne trematode infections.

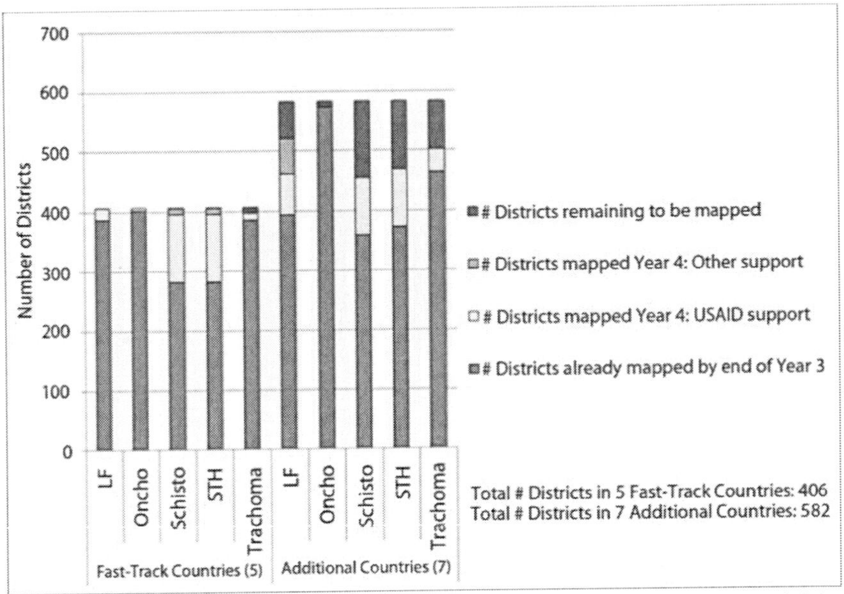

Source: Personal communication with USAID, Infectious Diseases Division, December 23, 2010.

Acronyms: lymphatic filariasis (LF), onchocerciasis (oncho), schistosomiasis (schisto), and soil-transmitted helminths (STH). These are the seven most common NTDs worldwide.

Note: The U.S. NTD Program began in 2006, therefore Years 3 and 4 refer to 2008 and 2009, respectively. Those countries that had earlier pilot programs and aimed at integrating disease-specific NTD control activities are called fast-track countries. These five countries (Burkina Faso, Ghana, Mali, Niger, and Uganda) could begin scaling up activities immediately. By the end of year three (2008), seven more countries were added. These additional countries were: Bangladesh, Cameroon, Haiti, Nepal, Sierra Leone, Sudan (southern region), and Togo.

Figure 2. Mapping of Seven Most Common NTDs in 12 Countries.

Of the 14 most common NTDs, roughly 80% are caused by STH—a group of three parasitic worms (roundworms, whipworms, and hookworms) that are contracted through contact with tainted soil or ingestion of eggs found on produce grown in tainted soil (*Figure 3*). More than 1 billion people are afflicted with STH worldwide, of whom children are the most vulnerable and tend to carry more than one type of worm at a time.

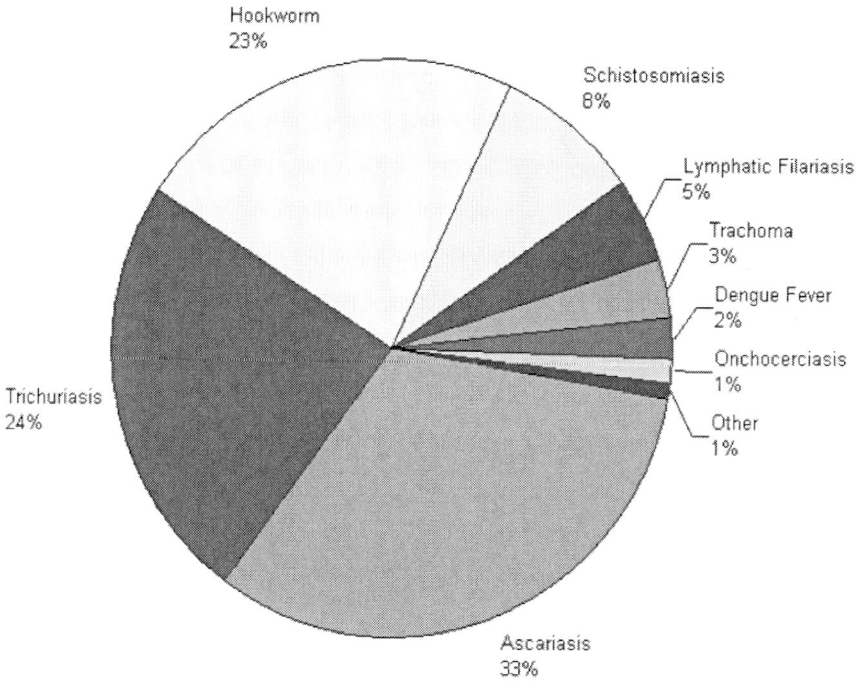

Source: Created by CRS from Peter Hotez, *Forgotten People, Forgotten Diseases* (Washington, DC: ASM Press, 2008), pp. 5, 106, and WHO, *Dengue and Dengue Haemorrhagic Fever*, Fact Sheet 117, March 2009.

Notes: Other includes leishmaniasis, Chagas disease, leprosy, sleeping sickness, Buruli ulcer, and guinea worm disease.

Figure 3. Prevalence of 12 Most Common NTDs.

NTDs independently cause high levels of illness and worsen the health of those plagued with other diseases like HIV/AIDS, malaria, and tuberculosis (TB). For example, some research indicates that

- **HIV/AIDS and schistosomiasis co-infection** is associated with higher HIV viral loads; people infected with schistosomiasis are more susceptible to HIV; and HIV-positive pregnant women who are co-infected with schistosomiasis have higher HIV-transmission rates than their counterparts without schistosomiasis;

- **malaria and STH co-infection** lead to higher incidence of anemia (a key cause of maternal and child mortality), and people with STH are more susceptible to malaria; and
- **TB and STH co-infection** is linked to higher rates of the conversion of latent TB into active TB, and TB vaccines are less effective in people co-infected with STH.

Of all global regions, sub-Saharan Africa is most affected by NTDs and by co-infection with HIV/AIDS, TB, and malaria co-infection (*Appendix E*).

CONTROL AND TREATMENT STRATEGIES

The international community has long sought to raise awareness about and support for tackling NTDs. In 1949, for example, world health leaders met to discuss schistosomiasis and noted the disease's harmful effects, especially its degenerative effect on economic development and food production.[7] Through ratification of several World Health Assembly resolutions through WHO and implementation of numerous public-private partnerships, the international community has agreed to prioritize combating, eliminating, and eradicating NTDs.[8] Well over 100 groups are engaged in fighting NTDs, including academia, the private sector, global development and health organizations, non-governmental organizations (NGOs), foundations, and national governments (*Table 2*). Some initiatives focus on one NTD, while others tackle a group of NTDs (*Appendix F*).

Among the 17 NTDs, 7 account for roughly 90% of the global NTD burden. These are the three soil-transmitted helminthes, schistosomiasis, lymphatic filiariasis, trachoma, and onchocerciasis. Drugs used to treat these seven diseases are donated by pharmaceutical companies or sold at subsidized prices ranging between \$0.02 and \$1.02, and are taken once or twice annually (depending on the concentration of the disease). At such prices, some 500 million people can be treated for these seven afflictions at roughly \$400 million annually.[9] When correctly used, these drugs can be used to control and, in some cases, eliminate some of the NTDs.[10]

Table 2. Key Stakeholders in NTD Control

Type of Partner	Key Roles
Recipient Governments	Development of integrated national plans, implementation, funding
Donor Governments	Funding, advocacy, technical assistance
International Organizations, especially WHO	Strategic direction, technical assistance, capacity building, drug procurement, monitoring and evaluation, disease surveillance, resource mobilization, donor coordination, advocacy
Philanthropic Organizations	Funding (grants), advocacy, and technical assistance
Pharmaceutical Companies	Research and development, drug donation and sales, logistics, research and development
Advocacy Groups	Advocacy and resource mobilization
Disease Based Initiatives	Assist national programs to implement NTD control, consensus building, resource mobilization
NGOs	Advocacy, financing, technical and operational support, implementation

Source: Summarized by CRS from the U.K. Department for International Development (DFID), DFID Support to the Control of Neglected Tropical Diseases: Review and Recommendations, 2009.

Historically, countries attempted to address each of these diseases in distinct programs. Within the past decade, WHO and other health experts found that national responses to these seven diseases could be integrated to improve the efficacy and reduce costs. Specifically, health experts found that

- medicines used to treat each of the seven NTDs could be safely administered to people co-infected with other NTDs (in most cases);
- one drug could treat more than one disease;
- individual diagnosis would not be necessary and entire communities could be safely treated, usually once per year, irrespective of each person's disease status;
- non-health workers, including teachers and community volunteers, could dispense the treatments in non-clinical settings (like schools) rather than in health facilities (which are often poorly resourced and in limited supply in remote areas); and
- the integration of drug delivery enabled resources to be pooled.

By integrating drug delivery for these seven diseases, countries and their partners have reduced some of the costs related to treating the diseases separately. After integrating mass drug administration (MDA) campaigns, USAID documented cost-efficiencies up to 41% and a 30% reduction in training costs.[11] USAID attributed these savings to streamlining program management, social mobilization, drug supply chains, and trainings.

The remaining 10 NTDs must be treated individually and can be more difficult and costly to manage. No cures exist for some of the NTDs in this group and for others available treatments can carry significant side effects. Additionally, access to diagnostic tools for some of these diseases may be limited, and treatment tends to be more costly because the medicines often need to be administered by trained health practitioners in health settings for prolonged periods. For some of these diseases, namely Chagas disease, dengue, human African trypanosomiasis, and leishmaniasis, early detection and treatment are vital to avoid irreversible disability or death.

Global NTD Plan

The global response to NTDs comprises complex mechanisms. Countries develop national NTD plans, primarily through the Ministries of Health and Education, and receive financial support from donors to help carry out the national MDA plans. WHO and donors like USAID review drug donation applications and support country-level planning, training, and monitoring and evaluation. Pharmaceutical companies provide treatments used for national NTD plans, either for free or at highly discounted rates. NGOs and faith-based organizations partner with national Ministries to implement the NTD plans. Academic groups, public-private partnerships, and pharmaceutical companies research and develop innovative treatments and control mechanisms.

In combating NTDs, countries and their supporters adhere to WHO protocols that outline best practices for addressing NTDs. In 2007, WHO released the *Global Plan to Combat Neglected Tropical Diseases*, which outlined several goals and targets for global control, elimination, and eradication of NTDs by 2015; strategic areas for action; and the policy framework for NTD implementation, monitoring, and evaluation.[12] Three key goals included in the plan were to

- eliminate or eradicate NTDs targeted in resolutions of the World Health Assembly and regional committees;
- reduce the burden of NTDs that can be treated with MDA; and
- ensure that interventions using novel approaches are available, promoted, and accessible for NTDs that are costly and difficult to treat.

As of October 2010, the WHO estimates that it would cost $1.7 billion to purchase enough drugs to treat all those at risk of contracting the seven most common NTDs. As of January 2010, donors had committed to provide all but one-third of the funds ($552 million) needed to fund the Global NTD Plan (*Table 3*). WHO estimates that it would cost an additional $1.2 billion to distribute the drugs.

ADVANCES IN TACKLING NTDS

In November 2010, WHO released its first report on NTDs. The report highlighted positive outcomes of long-standing efforts to tackle NTDs. The near eradication of dracunculiasis (guinea worm disease) is one of the most profound cases. Global incidence of guinea worm disease has declined 99% since 1986, when some 3.5 million people in Africa and Asia were infected. By 2009, only 3,190 cases were reported, and as of September 2010, WHO counted 1,613 cases (*Figure 4*).[13] Today, guinea worm disease is endemic in only four countries: Ethiopia, Ghana, Mali, and Sudan (accounting for about 90% of all cases). Prolonged conflict in Sudan has slowed efforts to eradicate guinea worm disease, though health experts remain optimistic about prospects that the illness could be the first infectious diseases to be eradicated since small pox in 1979.[14]

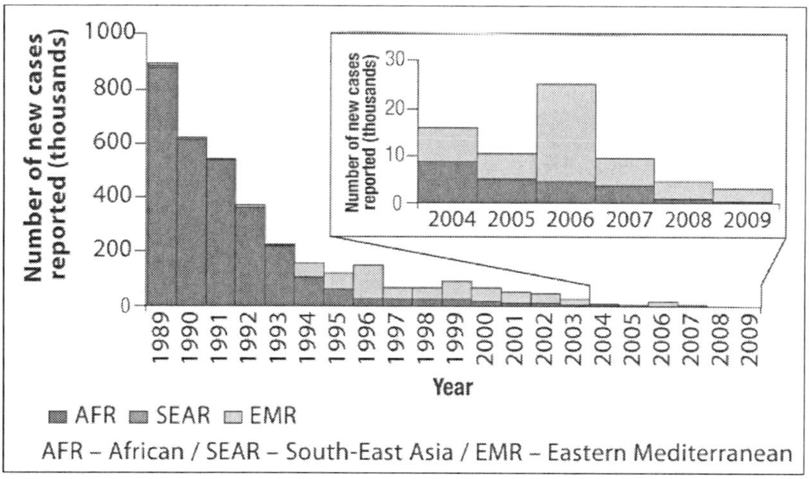

Source: WHO, First WHO Report on Neglected Tropical Diseases, 2010, p. 105.

Figure 4. Annual Incidence of Guinea Worm Diseases: 1989-2009.

Table 3. Need, Pledges, and Cost of Meeting Targets of the Global NTD Plan by 2015

Disease	Treatment	Needed Tablets (millions)	Total Pledged Tablets (millions)	Global Need Met (%)	Total Cost of Tablets (U.S. $ millions)	Per Capita Annual Cost of Tablets (U.S. $)
STH and LF	ALB	7,449	4,600	70%	124	0.02
Trachoma	AZI	1,690	500	30%	373	0.84
LF	DEC	7,248	7,300	63%	29	0.01
LF and	IVM					1.59
Oncho		1,967	1,967	100%	1,042	
Schisto	PZQ	1,942	100	5%	155	0.20
Trachoma	TZQ	19	not specified		3	0.33

Source: Compiled by CRS from personal communication with WHO, Neglected Tropical Diseases Department, October 22, 2010.

Notes: ALB can be substituted with MBD to treat STH at the same cost. The United States and Britain have pledged to provide up to 800 million PZQ tablets from 2011 to 2015. These pledges are not included in the table. Should these be included, the donations would be sufficient to meet the needs of nearly half of all people plagued with schistosomiasis.

Acronyms: Soil-Transmitted Helminths (STH), Lymphatic Filariasis (LF), Onchocerciasis (Oncho), schistosomiasis (Schisto), Albendazole (ALB), Azithromycin (AZI), Diethylcarbamazine (DEC), Ivermectin (IVM), Praziquantel (PZQ), and Tetracycline (TZQ).

Epidemiologists also celebrate advances in eliminating other NTDs. The Pan American Health Organization (PAHO), for example, reports that lymphatic filiariasis is no longer transmitted in three of seven Latin American countries where the disease was endemic.[15] Likewise, aggressive MDA campaigns have interrupted the transmission of onchocerciasis (river blindness) in one-third of areas where the disease was endemic and eliminated the disease from Columbia.[16] As such, people in 6 of the 13 previously endemic countries are no longer treated for the disease, and no new cases of onchocerciasis-related blindness have been reported in the region since 2007.[17]

U.S. Government Responses to NTDs

The United States has long supported efforts to control NTDs, and U.S.-based institutions, including the federal government, pharmaceutical companies, and philanthropic organizations, continue to lead global investments for and participation in fighting NTDs. Key U.S. government (USG) players include USAID, U.S. Centers for Disease Control and Prevention (CDC), National Institutes of Health (NIH), and Department of Defense (DOD). Non-profit and private sector participants include the Carter Center, the Bill & Melinda Gates Foundation, and several private companies, including Merck, Johnson & Johnson, and Pfizer. While each of these play a key role in combating NTDs, this report focuses on efforts conducted and supported by thc U.S. government.

In 2006, the U.S. government launched the Neglected Tropical Disease Control Program, its first effort to address a group of NTDs. The program was created in response to language in the FY2006 Foreign Operations Appropriations Act, which made available up to $15 million in "to support an integrated response to the control of neglected diseases including intestinal parasites, schistosomiasis, lymphatic filariasis, onchocerciasis, trachoma and leprosy."[18] The language signaled congressional support for calls to integrate and expand access to treatments against the seven most common NTDs. Until that time, most countries and their implementing partners focused on a single disease rather than targeting NTD co-infection. The NTD Program sought to document the feasibility of integrated NTD control and facilitate the advancement of this approach.

At the outset, the NTD program aimed to support the provision of 160 million NTD treatments to 40 million people through integrated programs in 15 countries. President George W. Bush reaffirmed his commitment to the program in 2008 and proposed spending $350 million from FY2008 through FY2013 on expanding the fighting against the seven NTDs to 30 countries.[19]

The NTD Program continues to be an important part of U.S. global health assistance under the Obama Administration. In May 2009, President Barack Obama announced the Global Health Initiative (GHI), which aims to streamline U.S. global health efforts. The President indicated that a key part of the initiative is to bolster support for U.S. efforts to combat NTDs and to integrate such efforts into other U.S. global health programs. The 2009-2014 Lantos-Hyde United States Government Malaria Strategy, for example, identifies plans to integrate malaria and NTD activities with other U.S. global health programs.[20] The Administration also intends to expand the provision of drugs that expel intestinal worms from children through USAID-supported education programs.

According to the Obama Administration, the NTD Program is part of a complete package of services the United States provides to improve the health of women, newborns, and children worldwide.[21] Through GHI, the Obama Administration set ambitious NTD targets in which the U.S. government would contribute to

- the administration of 1 billion NTD treatments;
- a 50% decrease in the prevalence of seven NTDs in 30 countries by 2013 that account for 70% of the global disease burden of the targeted diseases;
- the elimination of onchocerciasis in Latin America by 2016;
- the elimination of leprosy in all endemic countries by 2016; and
- the elimination of lymphatic filariasis globally by 2017.

As of September 30, 2010, the NTD Program had supported the provision of over 385 million treatments (*Figure 5*).[22] As of October 2010, USAID had identified 21 focus countries: Bangladesh, Burkina Faso, Cameroon, the Democratic Republic of Congo (DRC), Ethiopia, Ghana, Guinea, Haiti, Indonesia, Mali, Mozambique, Nepal, Niger, the Philippines, Uganda, Senegal, Sierra Leone, Sudan (southern region), Tanzania, Togo, and Vietnam.[23]

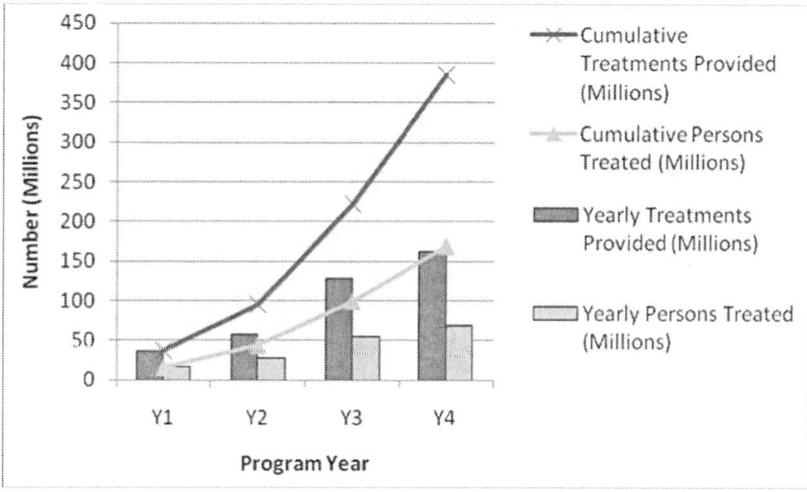

Source: Personal communication with USAID, Infectious Diseases Division, December 23, 2010. Notes: 2006 (Y1), 2007 (Y2), 2008 (Y3), 2009 (Y4).

Figure 5. NTD Treatments Distributed by USAID: 2006-2009.

U.S. Agency for International Development

USAID leads the NTD Program. In carrying out the program, USAID partners with foreign governments and other groups to bolster health systems, improve the capacity of the recipient countries to carry out NTD programs, coordinate donors' NTD efforts, and build political commitment to expand and sustain NTD programs.[24] Key functions of the NTD Program include the following:

- **Supporting national strategic planning**—USAID works with governments to develop and/or strengthen their national five-year NTD strategic plans. These efforts involve facilitating the coordination of ongoing donor efforts and bolstering country commitment to and ownership of programs.
- **Supporting implementation of NTD programs**—USAID provides technical and financial support to help countries achieve national coverage of integrated NTD programs. Related activities include disease mapping, securing drug donations, procuring non-donated NTD drugs (about 20% of NTD Program budget), training health

workers and community volunteers, strengthening supply chains and logistics management, and social marketing.

- **Monitoring and evaluation**—USAID supports efforts to measure the impact of NTD programs and develops models for integrating NTD projects into other global health efforts. The models focus on mapping disease prevalence, monitoring mass drug administration (MDA) campaigns to measure effectiveness and detect adverse effects, forecasting drug supplies, and tracking progress in meeting U.S. and global goals for disease elimination. To facilitate sharing of best practices, USAID publishes these finding and serves on several working groups with WHO and other partners.
- **Contributing to global guidelines and policies for NTD control**—USAID partners with WHO to share and refine tools, best practices, and lessons learned that have contributed to the refinement of global and regional standards for treating the seven most common NTDs. Some of the tools developed by USAID are now endorsed by WHO and are packaged as a standard "NTD Rollout Package" that countries use to establish or expand integrated NTD control.
- **Leveraging related USG programs**—where applicable, USAID leverages resources for programs related to malaria, education, water and sanitation, maternal and child health, and agriculture to NTD programs (e.g., offering deworming tablets in USAID-supported education programs).

U.S. Centers for Disease Control and Prevention

CDC focuses on the control and elimination of lymphatic filariais, onchocerciasis (river blindness), trachoma, schistosomiasis, and STH.[25] Through technical assistance to global partners and countries, CDC

- trains health workers, including ministry officials;
- conducts research for the development of tools to diagnose and combat NTDs, and to improve the integration of national NTD plans with other health interventions;
- supports mass drug administration for NTDs;
- supports monitoring and evaluation of MDA campaigns;
- develops global policy and guidelines for NTD programs; and

- studies NTDs not covered under the NTD Program to identify and develop tools and approaches to control and eliminate them.

National Institutes of Health

Several Institutes within NIH research tools to treat and eradicate NTDs. In FY2009, Congress provided $24 million to establish the Therapeutics for Rare and Neglected Diseases (TRND) program. The program applies expertise found across several Institutes to develop new candidate drugs for neglected diseases.[26] Additionally, the National Institute of Allergy and Infectious Diseases (NIAID) incorporates basic research on NTDs into several of its ongoing research efforts, including studies underway in the NIAID Laboratory on Parasitic Diseases and the Vector Biology Research Program, the Filariasis Research Reagent Repository Center, and the Schistosomiasis Resource Center. NIAID also participates in several public-private partnerships to develop new prevention and treatment options for NTDs. [27]

Department of Defense

The Department of Defense (DOD) has long recognized the detrimental effects of tropical diseases, especially in relationship to force protection.[28] Through collaborative agreements with the private sector and academia, for example, U.S. military infectious diseases programs played a significant role in the development of widely used vaccines, including those for yellow fever, mumps, measles, and polio. DOD also contributed to identifying the current dosing regimen for cutaneous leishmaniasisis and the vaccine for Japanese encephalitis.

Ongoing efforts related to NTDs, such as research for the development of a vaccine against dengue fever, are carried out in several DOD facilities, including eight infectious disease laboratories located around the world, animal laboratories, biosafety containment laboratories, a pilot vaccine facility, and clinical trials units.[29] Related DOD activities center on

- developing vaccines to prevent and drugs to treat infectious diseases;
- creating techniques to identify and diagnose infections rapidly;

- collecting and analyzing data to optimize infectious disease control strategies; and
- evaluating vector control methods.

CONGRESSIONAL ACTIONS TO ADDRESS NTDS

Since the November 2010 congressional elections, observers have speculated whether a change in House leadership and greater minority influence in the Senate might lead to reduced spending on foreign aid in general and global health in particular. However, bipartisan support for global health programs has remained strong in recent years, and interest in addressing NTDs has grown under both Republican and Democratic leadership. In 2008, Representative Donald Payne (D-NJ) and former U.S. Representative John Boozman (R-AR) launched the Congressional Malaria Caucus to raise congressional awareness about U.S. efforts to address malaria worldwide. In 2009, the Caucus added NTD control and prevention to its mission and became the Malaria and Neglected Tropical Diseases Caucus. U.S. Representatives Payne and Jeff Fortenberry (R-NE) will co-chair the caucus in the 112th Congress.

Congress has also demonstrated its support of controlling NTDs through steady increases in appropriations for addressing the diseases. From FY2006 through FY2010, Congress made available $135 million for NTD programs (*Table 4*). In each fiscal year between FY2006 and FY2008, Congress provided about $15 million to USAID for NTD programs. In FY2009, Congress made available $25 million for NTDs, some 67% higher than FY2008-enacted levels. Congress more than doubled appropriations for NTDs in FY2010, making available $65 million. The President requested $155 million for the NTD Program in FY2011. Congress has not yet enacted the FY2011 foreign operations appropriations, though the Senate Appropriations Committee reported out $100 million for NTD efforts (S. 3676). Congress did enact Continuing Appropriations and Surface Transportation Extensions Act, FY2011 (P.L. 111-322), which maintained funding for NTD programs at FY2010 levels through March 4, 2011.

Table 4. USAID and Department of State Global Health Spending: FY2006-FY2011 (current U.S. $ millions)

Program	FY2006 Actual	FY2007 Actual	FY2008 Actual	FY2009 Actual	FY2010 Actual	FY2006-FY2010 Total	FY2011 Request	Change FY2010-FY2011
CS/MH	447.8	427.9	521.9	651.0	681.6	2730.1	1058.0	55.2%
VC	29.7	19.6	20.5	30.5	18.4	118.7	18.1	-1.4%
HIV/AIDS	373.8	345.9	371.1	350.0	350.0	1790.8	350.0	0.0%
OID	445.1	586.4	707.9	781.4	1085.1	3605.8	1220.6	12.5%
TB	91.5	94.9	162.2	176.6	243.2	768.3	250.6	3.1%
Malaria	102.0	248.0	349.6	385.0	585.0	1669.6	680.0	16.2%
H5N1/H1N1	161.5	161.5	115.0	140.0	156.0	734.0	75.0	-51.9%
NTD	15.0	15.0	15.0	25.0	65.0	135.0	155.0	138.5.4%
Other	75.1	67.0	66.1	54.8	30.9	293.9	60.0	94.2%
FP/RH	435.0	435.6	457.2	552.4	650.6	2530.8	715.7	10.0%
Global Fund	247.5	247.5	0.0	100.0	0.0	595.0	0.0	0.0%
USAID Total	1,978.5	2,062.9	2,078.6	2,465.3	2,780.5	11,366.2	3,362.5	20.9%
State HIV/AIDS	1,771.1	2,869.0	4,116.4	4,559.0	4,609.0	17,930.5	4,800.0	4.1%
Global Fund	544.5	724.0	840.3	1,000.0	1,050.0	4,158.8	1,000.0	-4.8

Sources: Appropriations legislation and correspondence with USAID Budget Office.

Notes: Global Fund refers to the Global Fund to Fight AIDS, Tuberculosis, and Malaria, an international organization that combats the three diseases. The United States is the largest donor to this program.

KEY ISSUES RELATED TO NTD CONTROL

The term "neglected tropical diseases" describes a group of diseases with distinct characteristics. Some are easily treatable; others are not. Drugs can interrupt the transmission cycle of some NTDs, but treatments cannot eliminate others. The use of this term has helped to raise awareness about these long-standing health challenges, but it risks simplifying a complicated health challenge. Since all of these diseases are mostly rooted in poverty and the poor infrastructure that is usually found in destitute areas, the enduring solution to these illnesses is economic development. Industrialized countries, including the United States, have eliminated these diseases in their territories by combining drug treatment with the construction and use of latrines, modernization of agricultural practices, and utilization of improved water systems. Certainly, increased investments in NTD treatments have ameliorated the suffering of millions. More than 80% of NTDs, however, cannot be eliminated by drug delivery alone. As such, countries and their partners will need to indefinitely support the treatment of schistosomiasis and soil-transmitted helminths if complementary disease control methods are not applied.

In times of fiscal austerity, countries are re-evaluating their foreign assistance programs and seeking the most cost-efficient and effective approach to supporting international development. On January 19, 2011, USAID Administrator Rajiv Shah discussed the future of USAID and indicated that USAID would will increasingly consider the unit cost of impact when deciding which programs to fund or continue funding.[30] NTD control, through treatment alone, is one of the least expensive health interventions that the United States supports. It costs less than $2 annually to treat each person who needs to be treated for the seven most common NTDs that account for roughly 90% of all illnesses in this group. In contrast, the annual cost of first-line antiretroviral therapy for HIV/AIDS in sub-Saharan Africa averages about $95 per capita.[31] When antiretroviral treatments become less effective, the second-line treatments are considerably more expensive. These are not equally comparable, however, because HIV is always fatal if not treated, and only some NTDs are lethal when untreated. Also, HIV treatments must be taken daily, while treatments for the seven most common NTDs are usually taken once or twice annually. Nonetheless, both illnesses affect affected populations' capacity to live a productive life.

In FY2010, global HIV/AIDS programs and U.S. contributions to the Global Fund accounted for roughly 70% of all U.S. global health spending. In that fiscal year, U.S. support for NTDs amounted to less than 1% of the total global health budget. The section below explores key debates related to NTD control and includes a discussion on how Congress might address each of these arguments, which include the following:

- **Defining NTDs.** There is not yet a consensus on which diseases should be considered NTDs. WHO classifies 17 diseases, excluding HIV/AIDS, TB, and malaria, as NTDs. Yet some groups consider these three diseases to be neglected as well. With no agreement on which diseases constitute NTDs, investments in and analysis on this topic can be skewed and disjointed.
- **Evaluating reliance on MDA.** Although MDA campaigns have reduced disease prevalence and interrupted transmission, several limitations to MDA remain. For example, countries must have plans for continuing treatment after foreign aid ends, mismanagement and wider use of NTD treatments can result in disease resistance, and MDA does not interrupt transmission cycles of all NTDs.
- **Integrating development and health efforts and strengthening health information systems.** Depending on how development projects are implemented, they can exacerbate or decrease NTD infection rates. For instance, irrigation schemes could provide breeding grounds for vectors that spread NTDs, new transport infrastructure could facilitate the spread of parasites and vectors, and population resettlement may introduce parasite carriers to new areas.
- **Funding research and development (R&D).** Observers debate whether ongoing R&D efforts meet demands for NTD-related vaccines, treatments, and diagnostic tools. Specific concerns revolve around the toxicity and complicated regimens of some treatments, the absence of field-ready diagnostic tools for some NTDs, a lack of vaccines to prevent disease transmission, and vulnerability to drug resistance.

Defining "NTDs"

While experts agree that NTDs are long-standing health problems, cause chronic conditions, and have a high disease burden with low mortality, they do not agree on which diseases should be included in this list. Some health experts advocate an expansive list of diseases, while others promote concentrating resources on the seven most common and easily treated NTDs. In the 111th Congress, members of the Malaria and NTD Caucus urged USAID Administrator Rajiv Shah to develop a funding strategy for research and development of tools to treat, control, and eliminate leishmaniasis, Human African trypanosomiasis, and Chagas disease, which can be fatal if left untreated.[32] Supporters of expanding the definition also point to the threat some of these diseases could pose to the United States, particularly Chagas disease and dengue.[33]

Arguments against expanding the U.S. approach vary. Some fear that an overly expansive definition might diminish the gains made in raising support for countering these afflictions. Advocates of a concentrated approach, particularly on the seven most common NTDs, argue that these diseases should be eliminated or eradicated first to build momentum in sustained global health efforts. Additionally, when considering the full spectrum of NTDs, the seven most common NTDs are the least expensive to treat, increasing the likelihood that countries might sustain treatment campaigns, where necessary.

Defining NTDs: Issues for Congress

USAID leads U.S. efforts to combat NTDs, though other agencies and departments play a role in addressing the diseases (see "U.S. Government Responses to NTDs"). With the exception of language included in the FY2006 State, Foreign Operations appropriations,[34] Congress has not specified which neglected diseases the United States ought to address. Should Congress decide to do so, it could provide language defining NTDs through legislation similar to the Lantos-Hyde Act (P.L. 110-293), which outlines and authorizes the U.S. strategy to combating HIV/AIDS, TB, and malaria internationally. Alternatively, it could include such language in annual appropriations legislation.

Evaluating Reliance on Mass Drug Administration

Mass drug administration is at the heart of many NTD programs, including the U.S. NTD Program. In some cases, treating an entire population in an endemic area, irrespective of their disease status, has broken the transmission cycle of infection. In Latin America, for example, aggressive MDA campaigns have significantly reduced the disease burden of lymphatic filariasis. The Pan American Health Organization (PAHO) believes that transmission of the disease has been interrupted in three of seven endemic countries in the region.[35] Likewise, Merck, Inc., reports that onchocerciasis (river blindness) has been interrupted in one-third of areas formerly afflicted by the disease and that the disease has been eliminated from Colombia.[36]

There is debate, however, on the extent to which the United States should rely on this approach. A number of health analysts assert greater reliance on MDA might divert investments from strategies that could eliminate the diseases through more lasting measures, such as water and sanitation projects.[37] Observers are also concerned that prolonged use of MDA campaigns for diseases that cannot be eliminated with available medicines (such as soil-transmitted helminths and schistosomiasis that account for more than 80% of all NTDs) could hasten drug resistance. Scientists have already detected evidence of some disease resistance against treatments for hookworm, a soil-transmitted helminth.[38] Other health experts counter that these issues should not inhibit application of life-saving and health-enhancing measures that have led to the elimination of some NTDs. Additional issues at the heart of this debate include

- the capacity of countries to sustain MDA;
- the inability of MDA to break the transmission cycle of diseases such as STH; and
- application of preventive measures and disease surveillance.

Capacity to Sustain MDA

MDA has been used to advance efforts to eliminate some NTDs. Such progress, however, can be compromised if there is no effective long-term plan in place, particularly for NTDs like schistosomiasis and STH, which dwell in water and soil and have complicated life cycles that cannot be interrupted with MDA alone. In such cases, MDA campaigns must be sustained until the parasites are eliminated from the water or soil. At present, the U.S. NTD Program does not support vector management or other strategies that would interrupt the transmission of these diseases (such as latrine construction and improved water supply).

In Mali, for example, WHO and its partners launched a 10-year MDA campaign, which significantly reduced the prevalence of schistosomiasis. In 1992, the Malian government assumed full financial control of the program. The government was not able, however, to consistently procure drugs, maintain drug delivery, or reduce exposure of people to contaminated water.[39] Evaluators felt the treatment campaign that focused exclusively on schistosomiasis burdened the health system and diverted resources from routine health care.[40] After a decade of inconsistent MDA, prevalence rates had rebounded and reflected those seen before the campaign was initiated. In 2004, donors returned and supported the launch of another MDA campaign. This time, however, Mali and its partners launched an integrated treatment campaign that focused on more than one NTD and consolidated health management resources (see "Control and Treatment Strategies").

In addition to raising questions about the sustainability of some MDA programs, the Mali case also raises a long-standing debate about the extent to which donors should invest directly in health systems.[41] Some development organizations encourage the United States and other donors to reduce their reliance on contractors and channel more health assistance through local governments and organizations.[42] One official from the Ugandan Ministry of Health urges USAID to fully fund its NTD Program through the national health ministry rather than RTI International (an organization contracted to administer the U.S. NTD Program). He is concerned that the Ministry will not have the capacity to sustain the program once the financial support ceases since Ugandan stakeholders are not included in all aspects of project management and coordination.[43]

One study evaluating the first three years of the U.S. NTD Program, written in part by USAID officials, appears to contradict the assertion of the Ugandan official, indicating health system strengthening is an integral part of U.S. support. Specifically, the article highlights how resources provided through the NTD program were used to train more than 220,000 people, primarily community-based health workers and drug distributors, during the first three years of the program. The authors assert, "[t]raining is designed to empower these communities to treat NTDs within their own populations."[44]

Capacity to Sustain MDA: Issues for Congress

Several actions by the Obama Administration indicate an effort to enhance country ownership of global health programs. For example, country ownership has been highlighted as a key goal of the Global Health Initiative,[45] USAID Administrator Rajiv Shah has made public statements endorsing country ownership,[46] and the Office of the Global AIDS Coordinator (OGAC) advocates applying a "Partnership Framework" to HIV/AIDS programs funded through the President's Emergency Plan for AIDS Relief (PEPFAR).[47] The Partnership Framework outlines the role of the United States and recipient governments and describes how country ownership will ultimately assume full control of the programs. In Nigeria, for example, the government commits to funding half of the PEPFAR program by 2015.[48] According to one USAID official, key components of the NTD Program are to measure and document recipient country contributions to NTD responses; develop clear funding plans that outline the role of the donors and recipient country; and require commitments from participating countries to sustain and/or expand national financing of NTD control, including ensuring duty-free import of NTD drugs and dedicating at least one staff person to manage the NTD programs.[49]

Although USAID reportedly requires NTD focus countries to demonstrate political commitment to sustaining NTD plans, Congress might encourage or require the President to apply the Partnership Framework or similar approaches more broadly across all U.S. global health programs, including those aimed at NTDs and implemented in non-GHI or -NTD focus countries. Though it is too early to evaluate the Partnership Framework, the plan appears to include some of the processes that the Mali NTD program lacked: a clear strategy for preparing countries to assume full ownership of health projects, an outline of roles and responsibilities, alignment with national health plans, and investment in the national health system.

Several health and development experts argue that health systems of recipient countries must be strengthened if NTD programs supported by donors are to be sustained. One consortium of aid organizations recommends that donors allocate 15% of their budgets aimed at specific diseases to health system strengthening.[50] Should the 112th Congress support this idea, it could encourage or require that a portion of funds for the NTD Program (or other U.S. health programs like PEPFAR) be used on health system strengthening. The 112th Congress might also consider legislation similar to the Global HEALTH Act (H.R. 4933), which was introduced in the 111th Congress. The bill called for addressing some of the issues related to broad-based health training, and directed the President to develop a five-year global health strategy that emphasizes country ownership, integrated and coordinated U.S. global health assistance, and funding based on performance.

Other groups argue that concerns about the capacity of recipient countries to sustain NTD programs are unfounded for several reasons. First, donors are supporting plans developed largely by endemic countries. As such, countries receiving support have already prioritized and allocated some of their own resources to combating the diseases. Second, NTD treatment programs aimed at the seven most common NTDs pose little burden to health systems, as they can be administered by non-health workers (like teachers) outside of clinical settings. This community-based approach, some argue, bolsters weak health systems because it reaches people living in remote areas that usually have little access to health services, and increases demand for health services and awareness of health conditions in marginalized regions. Finally, budgets for treating the seven most common NTDs can be decreased as the diseases are eliminated. MDA cannot be independently applied to eliminate STH, however, which accounts for 80% of the NTD disease burden. Eggs from these parasites persist for years in soil, and the parasites can continue to thrive in other hosts, such as cattle.

Health Information Systems and Preventive Measures

NTDs are diseases of poverty. Strategies used to alleviate poverty can also help to prevent, eliminate, or eradicate these diseases. For example, development activities related to agricultural irrigation, dam construction, and forest clearance can facilitate the interruption of disease transmission. At the same time, if such projects are implemented without identifying disease prevalence through health impact assessments and integrating certain health measures, they can offer breeding grounds to several disease-carrying vectors, such as mosquitoes, and accelerate disease transmission.[51] Examples abound of development projects facilitating the spread of vector-born diseases. In Tanzania, for example, abandoned and poorly maintained sanitation projects have been identified as breeding grounds for mosquitoes carrying malaria or lymphatic filariasis.[52] Dam projects have led to the increase or introduction of schistosomiasis in Cameroon, Cote d'Ivoire, Ghana, Mali, Namibia, Senegal, and Sudan.[53]

Development experts need access to reliable data, however, to know where these diseases exist. Available data in most poor countries, however, are often outdated and based on small household surveys (see "Prevalence of Neglected Tropical Diseases"). If managers of large-scale development programs worked with health practitioners to ensure that disease prevalence surveys are conducted, then the inadvertent spread of disease during development projects could be avoided.[54] At the same time, health practitioners could gain a better understanding of disease prevalence, which could help in the planning, implementation, and monitoring of health initiatives.

The process of combating diseases through an approach that combines responses by practitioners across sectors, particularly those related to health, agriculture, water, construction, and waste disposal, is known as integrated vector management (IVM). WHO calls for a intersectoral approach to controlling NTDs that is based on five areas: MDA; intensified case-management; vector control; safe water, sanitation, and hygiene; and veterinary public health (that is, applying veterinary sciences to ensure the health and well-being of humans). Most countries, including the United States, that have successfully eliminated NTDs have utilized an IVM approach, particularly in the areas of water and sanitation.[55] Experts at the CDC assert that water and sanitation improvement should be a central component of any effective and sustainable approach to controlling NTDs.[56] One estimate indicates that improved sanitation and water safety can reduce the prevalence rates of schistosomiasis by 75% and blinding trachoma by 25%.[57] Water and sanitation improvement are particularly important when addressing pathogens that cannot be eliminated by drugs alone, such as STH and schistosomiasis.[58]

A comprehensive approach to NTD control might look like one that China is reportedly preparing to launch in sub-Saharan Africa. China is reportedly modeling the program after its own schistosomiasis control methods, which have led to interrupted transmission cycles in several regions across the country. The Chinese are reportedly planning to support the construction of latrines, the conversion of human and animal excrement into biofuel, and the procurement of tractors (to minimize contact with snail-infested water while farming).[59] Other examples of successful intersectoral approaches have included

- **collaboration among the health and agricultural sectors** in rice-growing regions of Asia to control malaria and Japanese encephalitis;[60]
- **collaboration among the health and agricultural sectors** to reduce the prevalence of soil-transmitted helminths in Korea;[61] and
- **collaboration among the health and housing sectors** to eliminate Chagas in Argentina.[62]

Health Information Systems and NTD Prevention: Issues for Congress

While arguments for improving health information systems often focus on determining when mass drug administration campaigns can be stopped and detecting disease resurgence, USAID also identified cost-efficiencies in improving these mechanisms. During the first two years of implementing the NTD Program, USAID purchased treatments for schistosomiasis according to country requested levels. USAID found, however, that countries did not always use prevalence data to estimate drug quantities or follow WHO treatment guidelines. This led to inefficiencies, including drug overstocks in some areas and shortages in others. In the third year, USAID developed a new procurement system that improved drug management and forecasting processes. After improving the drug management system, USAID found that fewer drugs needed to be procured.[63]

Observers maintain cost-efficiencies can also be found by better integrating NTD programs with other health programs. Proponents assert the community networks that provide NTD drugs could also distribute insecticide-treated bednets and treatments against HIV/AIDS, TB, and malaria. Conversely, bednets used in malaria programs could also help to prevent people from contracting lymphatic filariasis.[64] The Lantos-Hyde United States Government Malaria Strategy identifies plans to integrate malaria and NTD activities but does not specify how this will occur.

Improved integration of NTD activities into projects funded through the Senator Paul Simon Water for the Poor Act (P.L. 109-121) may present another opportunity to intensify NTD control.[65] The Act authorized the President to develop an integrated strategy for improving water and sanitation worldwide. According to a 2010 report to Congress, the Administration has developed strategies for 34 countries, which include all NTD focus countries.[66] The United States might also consider sharing resources provided through the Millennium Challenge Corporation (MCC) for water and sanitation programs. Although MCC water programs tend to emphasize reducing diarrheal-related deaths, populations suffering from diarrhea are often afflicted with other water-borne diseases like schistosomiasis (though the diseases may not be detected).

Observers have cited instances in which U.S. aid agencies operating in the same country have used different implementing partners, consulted with different stakeholders when planning the projects, and partnered with different government officials, even when focusing on the same health challenge. While acknowledging duplication in some areas of U.S. health aid, Secretary of State Hillary Clinton contended GHI aims to address this challenge.[67] Nonetheless, with little available documentation on GHI, not much is known on the extent to which the initiative is curbing such practices. USAID also maintained these criticisms do not apply to U.S.-supported NTD programs because they support national NTD plans.[68] Where possible, ambassadors in recipient countries could ensure that USG agencies implementing health and development projects operate from joint working agreements and align their activities (including training, reporting, funding, and target populations), especially in non-GHI focus countries.[69] The 2010 Quadrennial Diplomacy and Development Review appears to endorse this idea.

Funding Research and Development of Innovative Tools

Widespread use of the term NTD belies the complexity of the health challenge. The existence, efficacy, and availability of tools to diagnose, cure, and control each disease vary. Progress in controlling, eliminating, and eradicating NTDs also varies among the geographical locations. The seven most common NTDs that account for 90% of all NTD cases can be treated with relatively inexpensive drugs that are effective in low-resource settings. Through massive treatment programs, two of these seven diseases, onchocerciasis and lymphatic filariasis, have been nearly eliminated in some settings. People living in areas endemic with two other NTDs (schistosomiasis and STH) that account for 80% of all NTD cases, however, must be treated indefinitely if other public health measures are not taken (e.g., building and using latrines and ensuring proper use of purified water). Other NTDs, like dengue and buruli ulcer, have no known cure. Another NTD, human African trypanosomiasis (sleeping sickness), is always fatal if not treated; another, leishmaniasis, is treated with drugs that are extremely toxic and difficult to administer. To address these challenges, several health advocates call for greater investments in R&D in four key areas:

- **Drug and vaccine development**—While donor funding has led to an unprecedented capacity to treat NTDs, some analysts are concerned about drug resistance and urge prudence in drug administration, particularly for diseases that cannot be eliminated through MDA. Others argue that these concerns should not hinder the provision of drugs that alleviate human suffering and save lives. Several experts also call for researchers to develop vaccines that can prevent people from contracting NTDs and to create innovative treatments for diseases with no cure, or for which available drugs are toxic or carry complicated regimens (both in terms the complexity of administering the medicine and the duration of treatment).
- **Vector Control**—For most NTDs, there are no vaccines to prevent infection and MDA programs cannot independently eradicate the pathogen. In such circumstances, vector control often plays a vital role. However, several peer-reviewed articles highlight challenges related to vector control, including growing pesticide resistance caused in part by improper application or overuse.
- **Diagnostic Tools**—Disease monitoring and surveillance are critical for detecting drug resistance and treatment-related complications,

identifying interruptions in disease transmission, determining when MDA can be ceased, and identifying disease resurgence (especially after a disease has been eliminated). However, available diagnostic tools may not be useful in low-resource settings that lack sufficient quantities of laboratory equipment and trained health practitioners. As such, some epidemiologists are concerned that poorer countries may not be able to assume full control of disease surveillance tasks.

- **Operational Research**—Some health experts encourage further consideration of factors that might affect drug efficacy or safety, such as co-application of traditional remedies and treatments for HIV/AIDS, TB, and malaria.[70] Some evidence indicates, for example, that the vaccine against TB is less effective among people infected with schistosomiasis.[71] More research could also be useful to study the impact of NTD treatments on those infected with other NTDs. Researchers found, for example, that people co-infected with onchocerciasis and loaisis should not be treated with a drug (ivermectin) commonly used to cure onchocerciasis, as they could experience serious side effects or death.[72] Observers also call greater attention to factors related to NTDs that are more complicated to treat, such as maintaining drug efficacy without refrigeration. These issues buttress calls for bolstering research and development in developing countries, particularly in sub-Saharan Africa.

The weak medicine regulatory authorities (MRAs) in several developing countries also warrant consideration.[73] In order to ensure the safety and efficacy of a proposed drug, MRAs need access to fully functioning laboratories and well-trained technicians capable of testing samples and determining whether medicines meet quality criteria. In a 2007 WHO study, almost all high-income countries reported having a quality management system in place to monitor adverse drug reactions (ADRs), while only 50% of low-income countries reportedly evaluated medicines to detect ADRs.[74] Without the resources to evaluate properly the safety, efficacy, and quality of new medicines, one team of experts found that MRAs in most low-income countries, particularly in Africa, rely heavily on MRAs in high-income countries. For NTD treatments, however, regulatory authorities in high-income countries may not have sufficient safety and efficacy data on which to conduct comprehensive risk-benefit assessments when approving drugs intended for poorer countries and may not consider complications that are pervasive in poorer areas.

Funding Research and Development: Issues for Congress

According to a study conducted by the George Institute for International Health, the United States is the world's largest funder of research and development for the treatment and control of NTDs (*Table 5*).[75] In FY2008, the USG accounted for roughly 41% of all funding for NTD-related R&D and about 48% of all spending by the top 12 donors. If contributions by the Bill & Melinda Gates Foundation are added, total U.S. support for R&D for NTDs accounted for 62% of all spending and 71% of outlays by the top 12 donors. Nonetheless, NTD activists call for greater investments in NTD research, particularly since HIV/AIDS, TB, and malaria accounted for 72% of these funds in 2008 (*Table 6*). Some analysts believe that investments in these diseases outpace spending on other NTDs, because high-income countries are also susceptible to and affected by HIV/AIDS and TB.

The U.S. government has demonstrated support for higher spending on R&D for global health overall and for NTDs in particular. In a March 2010 letter to USAID Administrator Shah, several members of Congress called on USAID to determine an appropriate funding strategy that considers R&D funding for NTDs.[76] The Agriculture, Rural Development, Food and Drug Administration, and Related Agencies Appropriations Act, Fiscal Year 2010 directed the FDA to establish internal review groups to address rare and neglected diseases, to report to Congress one year after establishing the review groups and to issue guidance relating to rare and neglected diseases.[77] In March 2010, the Food and Drug Administration (FDA) established two new expert working groups, the Rare Disease Review Group and the Neglected Disease Review Group.[78] In September 2010, the neglected diseases group hosted a public hearing to share ideas with stakeholders on how FDA should tackle neglected diseases. The Neglected Disease Review Group is expected to submit a report to Congress that includes recommendations on how FDA should address NTDs. Ahead of the findings, the FDA has already indicated that it needs additional resources to provide training and hire additional staff with expertise in NTDs.[79]

Table 5. Spending on NTD Research and Development, 2007 and 2008 (millions and %)

Donor	2007			2008		
	Current U.S. $	% of Top 12 Donors	% of Total R&D Funding	Current U.S. $	% of Top 12 Donors	% of Total R&D Funding
U.S. National Institutes of Health	1,064.9	46.6%	41.6%	1,119.6	41.6%	36.2%
Bill & Melinda Gates Foundation	452.1	19.8%	17.7%	640.4	23.8%	20.7%
Drug and Biotechnology Companies	231.9	10.2%	9.1%	390.2	14.5%	12.6%
European Commission	121.4	5.3%	4.7%	145.7	5.4%	4.7%
U.S. Agency for Int. Development	80.6	3.5%	3.1%	87	3.2%	2.8%
U.S. Department of Defense	86.9	3.8%	3.4%	75.3	2.8%	2.4%
The Wellcome Trust	60	2.6%	2.3%	60.4	2.2%	2.0%
U.K. Medical Research Council	51.7	2.3%	2.0%	52.4	1.9%	1.7%
U.K. Department for Int. Development	47.6	2.1%	1.9%	43	1.6%	1.4%
Dutch Ministry of Foreign Affairs	33.9	1.5%	1.3%	30.2	1.1%	1.0%
Institut Pasteur	31.6	1.4%	1.2%	29.8	1.1%	1.0%
Sweden Int. Development Agency	21.5	0.9%	0.8%	20.5	0.8%	0.7%
Subtotal of Top 12 Donors	2,284.1	100.0%	89.2%	2,694.5	100.0%	87.1%
Total R&D Funding	2,560.1			3,094.2		

Source: The George Institute for International Health, *Neglected Disease Research & Development: New Times, New Trends*, December 2009, p. 67.

Table 6. Spending on R&D for Health Products to Be Applied in Developing Countries, by Disease, 2007 and 2008 (millions and %)

Disease	2007 Current U.S. $	2007 Share of Funding	2008 Current U.S. $	2008 Share of Funding
HIV/AIDS	1,083.0	42.3%	1,215.8	39.3%
Malaria	468.4	18.3%	566.0	18.3%
Tuberculosis	410.4	16.0%	467.5	15.1%
Kinetoplastids	125.1	4.9%	145.7	4.7%
Diarrhea	113.9	4.4%	138.1	4.5%
Dengue	82.0	3.25	132.5	4.3%
Pneumonia & Meningitis	32.5	1.35	96.1	3.1%
Helminth Infections	51.6	2.0%	69.5	2.3%
Salmonella	9.1	0.4%	41.1	1.3%
Leprosy	5.6	0.2%	10.1	0.3%
Rheumatic Fever	1.7	0.1%	2.3	0.1%
Trachoma	1.7	0.1%	2.2	0.1%
Buruli Ulcer	2.4	0.1%	2.1	0.1%
Platform Technologies	10.0	0.4%	16.6	0.6%
Core funding of a Multi-Disease R&D Organization	110.9	4.3%	110.4	3.4%
Unspecified Disease	51.6	2.0%	78.2	2.5%
Grand Total	2,560.0	100.0%	3,094.2	100.0%

Source: The George Institute for International Health, *Neglected Disease Research & Development: New Times, New Trends*, December 2009, p. 15.

Note: Kinetoplastid parasites cause disease in humans, animals and plants, severely affecting human health and retarding agriculture development in less developed countries. Sleeping sickness, Chagas disease, and leishmaniases are the major human diseases caused by kinetoplastids. NTDs are bolded.

Congress has also authorized market incentives to encourage R&D on NTDs. The Orphan Drug Act of 1983 (P.L. 97-414) and the Rare Diseases Orphan Product Development Act (ODA) of 2002 (P.L. 107-281), for example, offer tax credits, market exclusivity, and priority review vouchers. Despite these actions, relatively few innovative NTD products have been developed. One study indicated that between 1983 and 2008, the FDA approved 325 orphan drug products, two of which were for NTDs. One expert at the Center for Global Development contended that all of the NTD products that were developed "had limited or no value because their formulation and pricing were inappropriate for developing country settings."[80] Some health analysts have contended that major pharmaceutical companies have produced a limited number of NTD products because the low profit margins (if any) of NTD products leave little incentive to invest in R&D.[81]

In response to relatively low spending levels on NTD R&D by larger pharmaceutical companies, some advocates call for enhancing R&D capacity in developing countries and supporting public-private partnerships that include specialists from poorer countries. Innovative partnerships with experts hailing from endemic areas have reportedly developed tools that were cheaper and better adapted for field use.[82] Some proponents call for boosting U.S. funding for consortiums such as the Special Program for Research and Training in Tropical Diseases (TDR) and the Drugs for Neglected Diseases *initiative* (DND*i*), which have played a critical role in identifying innovative NTD tools.[83] The $4.8 million the United States donated to TDR during the 2008-2009 budget period amounted to about 6% of all contributions.[84] The $1.4 million the United States contributed to DND*i* accounted for 0.9% of all donations.[85]

In addition to calls for greater U.S. support for NTD-related R&D, supporters urge the 112th Congress to consider enacting legislation similar to a bill introduced in the 111th Congress called the 21st Century Global Health Technology Act (111th Congress, H.R. 3560/S. 1591), which would have authorized $5 million in each fiscal year from 2010 through 2014 to improve laboratory capabilities in developing countries. Other recommendations for encouraging companies to develop drugs for the poor and strengthening medicine regulatory capacity in low-income countries include

- aligning U.S. regulatory guidelines with those of the WHO;
- encouraging pharmaceutical companies to use and develop patent pools;

- including regulators from endemic areas when conducting regulatory reviews of novel NTD products; and
- applying U.S. regulatory expertise to the review of novel NTD products produced outside the United States.

FINAL DISCUSSION

As noted, neglected tropical diseases are diseases that primarily plague the poorest people in the poorest parts of the world. Changes in the environment and population flows, however, make industrialized countries, including the United States, vulnerable to some NTDs as well. In May 2009, CDC reported that 28 people who lived or had visited Key West, FL, had contracted dengue.[86] With the exception of a few dengue cases that occurred along the Texas-Mexico border in the 1990s, the Florida Keys cases were the first dengue cases reported in the continental United States since 1946.[87] Some observers are concerned that mosquitoes capable of spreading dengue fever are gradually spreading across the United States, particularly since there is no vaccine or treatment against this disease. Without the care of trained physicians, about 20% of those infected with dengue haemorrhagic fever (DHF) die. Access to health practitioners who are trained to identify DHF and treat its effects can reduce that rate to about 1%. Mosquitoes capable of spreading dengue are now found across the southeastern United States, along the eastern seaboard up to southern New England, and around areas bordering the Mississippi River and its watershed up to Chicago. Scientists expect the mosquitoes to broaden their range.[88]

In recent years, cases of Chagas have also emerged within the continental United States (thought by some to have been brought by migrants from Latin America). While blood centers are now required to test for Chagas,[89] some health experts surmise that several cases remain undiagnosed in the United States and that Chagas stands as an undetected cause of heart disease and stroke.[90] In addition, travelers from industrialized countries are increasingly contracting NTDs like schistosomiasis, while engaged in eco-tourism and other travel "off the beaten track." These cases are usually identified once tourists develop severe, acute infection or other unusual problems.[91]

Concerns about domestic vulnerability to NTDs bolster the view that improving global health and countering NTDs is mutually beneficial for recipient and donor countries. While poor countries could benefit from U.S. research and development of innovative tools to treat and detect NTDs, for example, the United States could be better protected by an improved capacity to detect and respond to emergent cases of tropical diseases within its borders. The 112th Congress might consider introducing a bill similar to one that the House passed in the 111th Congress that calls for the Secretary of the Department of Health and Human Services to report to Congress on "the epidemiology of, impact of, and appropriate funding required to address neglected diseases of poverty." Included among the diseases specified in the bill are Chagas and soil-transmitted helminths.[92]

The United States offers more resources to tackle NTDs than any other country. The U.S. approach to addressing this problem, however, faces several complicating factors. These include the following:

Conflict—When conflict erupts, treatment programs are frequently interrupted, which provides the disease an opportunity to resurge. Additionally, NTDs can easily spread in the crowded and sometimes unsanitary conditions of refugee camps.[93]

Global urbanization—Trends indicate that by 2050, 75% of the world's populations will live in urban areas. Much of this growth is expected to occur in poor countries already struggling to meet the basic needs of their populations. Unfettered population shifts from rural to urban areas coupled with poor urban planning could lead to increased NTD outbreaks in urban areas. People carrying soil-transmitted helminths, for example, could move to urban areas and spread the disease, particularly in slums where access to clean water, sanitation, and health services is limited.[94]

Other donor support—Efforts by philanthropy groups and pharmaceutical companies aside, few donors have pledged to provide sufficient resources to fund NTD-related resolutions (though they may be engaged in bilateral efforts).[95] At the 2008 G8 summit, Members committed to support global NTD efforts and to reach at least 75% of people infected with NTDs.[96] Following the summit, Britain pledged to spend £50 million (about $92 million in 2008) over five years to combat NTDs, and the United States announced its plan to spend $350 million on NTDs over five years (see "U.S. Government Responses to NTDs").[97] Additionally, in May 2010, the Netherlands pledged to provide up to €70 million (about $87 million) over four years for the development of medicines and vaccines against several diseases, including NTDs.[98]

Some groups call for countries like Brazil, China, and India to contribute more to the global fight against NTDs, especially since they have received financial assistance to address NTDs and their economies have demonstrated strong growth. One study indicates that the global disease burden for soil-transmitted helminths, lymphatic filariaisis, and trachoma could be reduced by 20% if Brazil, China, India, and Russia assumed full control over their own NTD control and elimination efforts.[99] This assertion is particularly provocative, as one report discusses the emergent role of Brazil, China, India, Russia, and South Africa in addressing global health challenges worldwide.[100] Similarly, one expert calls on the Organization of Islamic Conference to contribute to the Global NTD Plan, particularly since member countries including Bangladesh, Chad, Mali, Niger, Nigeria, Indonesia, Somalia, Sudan, and Yemen, all have NTDs.[101]

Veterinary Capacity—WHO and other experts express concern about limited expertise in addressing NTDs in some countries and declining knowledge in others, particularly in the areas of vector control, case-management, pesticide management and veterinary health. Since some NTDs are zoonotic infections—human infections originating in animals—monitoring and controlling the diseases in animals are critical and often overlooked parts of NTD control. WHO recommends a five-pronged approach to tackling NTDs, which includes strengthening veterinary capacity.[102]

At a January 2011 speech, USAID Administrator Shah indicated the agency would increasingly make tough decisions while considering which health and development efforts to fund. Specifically, the unit cost of impact would be the key determinant. Measuring the cost effectiveness of health programs could be a complicated endeavor. For example, what factors should be weighed more heavily: mortality rates, disease prevalence, or contagiousness? How might the United States address diseases that countries might not prioritize, but could be easily spread? Should countries receive assistance based on their ability to fund a national response or based on their portion of the global disease burden?

For NTDs in particular, several other questions might arise. How might countries graduate from U.S. health assistance if NTDs that cause more than 80% of the NTD disease burden cannot be eliminated by treatment alone and affected countries have several other health challenges to consider? If the United States reduces support for a more expensive health issue, like HIV/AIDS, would countries maintain less expensive programs that carry a lower mortality rate like NTDs? While there appears to be consensus on the need to reevaluate U.S. foreign assistance programs, experts do not yet agree on the best approach to this challenging exercise.

APPENDIX A. ACRONYMS

ADR	Adverse drug reaction
ALB	Albendazole
AZI	Azithromycin
CDC	U.S. Centers for Disease Control and Prevention
DEC	Diethylcarbamazine
DHF	Dengue Haemorrhagic Fever
DND*i*	Drugs for Neglected Diseases *initiative*
DoD	Department of Defense
FDA	U.S. Food and Drug Administration
GHI	Global Health Initiative
IVM	Ivermectin
LF	Lymphatic Filariasis
MCC	Millennium Challenge Corporation
MDA	Mass Drug Administration
MRA	Medicine regulatory authority
NIAID	National Institute of Allergy and Infectious Diseases
NIH	National Institutes of Health
NGO	Non-Governmental Organization
NTD	Neglected Tropical Disease
ODA	Rare Diseases Orphan Product Development Act
OGAC	Office of the Global AIDS Coordinator
Oncho	Onchocerciasis
PAHO	Pan American Health Organization
PEPFAR	President's Emergency Plan for AIDS Relief
PZQ	Praziquantel
R&D	Research and Development
Schisto	Schistosomiasis
STH	Soil-Transmitted Helminths
TB	Tuberculosis
TZQ	Tetracyclilne
USAID	U.S. Agency for International Development
USG	U.S. Government
WASH	Water, sanitation, and hygiene
WHO	World Health Organization

APPENDIX B. GLOSSARY

Anemia—abnormally low hemoglobin concentration in the blood. Hookworm, for example, can cause iron deficiency anemia or loss of iron in the blood.

Chemotherapy—the use of chemicals or antibiotics to treat an infection, a malignancy, or other condition with the aim of curing it or preventing its further progress.

Coverage—the proportion of people in a target population or group who have taken a drug or drug combination.

Disability-adjusted life years—a measure of overall disease burden, expressed as the number of years lost due to ill-health, disability, or early death.

Disease burden—the amount of ill health from a given cause (disease, injury, cause of disease, or risk factor) in a population of interest.

Disease mapping—a method for displaying spatial distribution of cases of disease.

Elimination—the control of a previously prevalent communicable disease by reducing case transmission to a predetermined low level, although not necessarily to zero. The aim is to achieve a situation where the infecting agent cannot sustain itself in the population until the disease no longer presents a major public health problem.

Endemic—the constant presence in a population of a condition such as a communicable disease.

Eradication—ending all transmission of an infectious disease agent by bringing about the extermination of the disease agent. Diseases such as guinea worm, measles, and polio have been eradicated regionally. Smallpox, however, is the only disease to have been eradicated globally.

Incidence—the occurrence of new disease events or cases.

Incidence rate, the rate at which new events occur in a population.

Infectious disease—an illness due to a specific agent or its toxic products that arises through transmission of that agent or its products from an infected person, animal, or reservoir to a susceptible host, either directly or indirectly through an intermediate plant or animal host, vector, or the inanimate environment.

Integrated Vector Management—a decision-making process for the management of vector populations, so as to reduce or interrupt transmission of vector-borne diseases. An integrated vector management approach takes into account the available health infrastructure and resources and integrates all available and effective measures across all sectors.

Mass drug administration—delivery of a preventive or therapeutic regimen to the entire population or to selected portions of it.

Morbidity—sickness, the state or condition of being unwell. **Morbidity rate** measures the proportion of people who have become sickened by a particular disease over a given time period (usually measured annually). Also, **incidence rate.**

Mortality—death. **Mortality rate**—measures the proportion of people who have died from a given cause within a certain time (usually measured annually).

Pathogen—an organism that causes disease.

Prevalence—the total number of designated conditions, such as cases of a disease or patterns of behavior, that are present in a population at a point in time, regardless of the duration of time for which the condition or disease has been experienced by individuals in the population.

Reservoir—a receptacle for storage. *Reservoir of infection*, for example, refers to human or animal hosts of infectious pathogens.

Second-line treatment—offered to patients when initial therapy (first-line treatment) fails.

Vector—a living creature, usually an insect, that carries an infectious pathogen to a susceptible human host.

Appendix C. NTDs: Prevalence, Characteristics, and Regional Distribution

Disease	Prevalence (million)	Population at Risk (millions)	Regions of Highest Prevalence	Reservoir	Mode of Transmission	Symptoms	Treatment Availability and Cost
Buruli Ulcer	0.05	Unknown	Sub-Saharan Africa	Unknown, fauna, flora, and other ecological aspects of the wetlands suspected	Experts are uncertain, but evidence suggests the germ enters the body through the skin at a site of trauma. Insects may also be natural reservoirs and their bites could transmit the disease to humans. Environmental changes that promote flooding, such as deforestation, dam construction, and irrigation systems, are often associated with Buruli ulcer outbreaks. Population increases in rural wetlands also raise exposure to the disease.	Big ulcers and severe scarring, resulting in disfiguration and sometimes loss of limbs	Treatment is more expensive as the disease progresses. If treated early, medication costs roughly $38. Best estimates indicate that the average cost of treatment and surgery reach $780 per capita in the advanced stages.

Appendix C. (Continued).

Disease	Prevalence (million)	Population at Risk (millions)	Regions of Highest Prevalence	Reservoir	Mode of Transmission	Symptoms	Treatment Availability and Cost
Chagas disease	16-18	100	United States, Latin America and Caribbean	Humans and large blood sucking insects known as "kissing bugs"	Chagas disease is transmitted by the infected feces of blood-sucking bugs called triatomine. After biting humans, the bug usually defecates near the site. The parasites enter the body when the person smears (usually while scratching) the bug feces into the bite, eyes, mouth, or any skin break. Chagas disease is also transmitted by: ingestion of food contaminated with the feces of the bug, blood transfusion or organ transplantation, or mothers during delivery or pregnancy.	Cardiac complications, including heart disease or failure; intestinal complications; enlarged esophagus or colon; or swelling internal organs	Treatment options are limited if not addressed in the early stages. Best estimates indicate that the average annual cost of treating chronic Chagas is $1,028.

Appendix C. (Continued).

Disease	Prevalence (million)	Population at Risk (millions)	Regions of Highest Prevalence	Reservoir	Mode of Transmission	Symptoms	Treatment Availability and Cost
Dengue	50	2,500	United States, tropical, and sub-tropical areas	Mosquito	Bite of infective mosquito.	Fever, headache, rash, and intense pain. Untreated, dengue fever (an advanced form of dengue) is fatal 20% of the time. The mortality rate can be reduced to about 1% with care from trained health workers.	None, trained physicians can mitigate related symptoms.
Dracunculiasis (guinea worm)	0.01	Unknown	Sub-Saharan Africa	Humans	Ingestion of larvae found in stagnant fresh water.	Intense pain, blisters, ulcers, fever, and vomiting	None, surgery to remove the worms.

Appendix C. (Continued).

Disease	Prevalence (million)	Population at Risk (millions)	Regions of Highest Prevalence	Reservoir	Mode of Transmission	Symptoms	Treatment Availability and Cost
Fascioliasis	17	Unknown	Worldwide	Humans, cattle, and snails	Ingesting water or uncooked aquatic plants (such as watercress) contaminated with snail larvae.	Hemorrhage, fibrosis of the liver, growth deficiencies; abdominal pain, respiratory problems; and skin rashes.	Tablets are taken once or twice annually and are donated free of charge by drug manufacturers. Should demand exceed the donated amounts, drugs can be purchased for between $0.32 and $1.02 per person.

Appendix C. (Continued).

Human African trypanosomiasis (sleeping sickness)	0.3	60	Sub-Saharan Africa	Humans, though the role of domestic and wild animals is not clear	The bite of infective tsetse flies that contract the parasite from infected humans and animals. Once infected, a tsetse fly remains infective for life (between 3 months and 10 months). Transmission from blood transfusion and contaminated medical products is possible.	Fever; swollen lymph glands; aching muscles and joints; headaches; damage to the central nervous system, causing changes in personality, confusion, slurred speech, seizures, and impaired walking and talking	According to WHO, pharmaceutical donations reportedly meet all needs as expressed by affected countries. Sleeping sickness is always fatal if not treated.
Leishmaniasis (kala azar)	14	350	United States, former Soviet states, south/ southwestern Asia; Mexico, South and Central America; sub-Saharan Africa and Australia	Humans and locally variable wildlife including, rodents, sloths, marsupials, and dogs	The bite of infective sandflies that contract the parasite from infected mammals and through blood transfusion, in rare cases.	Skin ulcers and lesions, destruction of the mucous membranes, fever, swelling of the spleen and liver, and anemia	According to WHO, treatments cost between $110 and $600.

Appendix C. (Continued).

Disease	Prevalence (million)	Population at Risk (millions)	Regions of Highest Prevalence	Reservoir	Mode of Transmission	Symptoms	Treatment Availability and Cost
Leprosy	0.2	Unknown	India; Latin America and Caribbean; and sub-Saharan Africa	Humans and armadillos in Louisiana and Texas	Unknown. Leprosy transmission is favored by close contact. Some scientists believe leprosy is transmitted from the nasal mucosa of an infected individual to the skin and respiratory tract of another person.	Nerve damage, muscle weakness, atrophy, and permanent disability	According to WHO, pharmaceutical donations reportedly meet all needs as expressed by affected countries.
Lymphatic filariasis (elephantiasis)	120	1,300	East and South Asia; Pacific Islands; and sub-Saharan Africa	Humans. In Asia, cats, civets, and non-human primates.	Bite of a mosquito harboring infective larvae.	In the late stages, painful, disfiguring swelling of the legs and genital organs	Tablets are taken once or twice annually and are donated free of charge by drug manufacturers. Should demand exceed the donated amounts, drugs can be purchased for between \$0.05 and \$0.10 per person.

Appendix C. (Continued).

Disease	Prevalence (million)	Population at Risk (millions)	Regions of Highest Prevalence	Reservoir	Mode of Transmission	Symptoms	Treatment Availability and Cost
Onchocerciasis (river blindness)	37	90	Latin America and Caribbean; and sub-Saharan Africa	Humans and in gorillas (rarely)	Bite of an infected female blackfly that contracts the disease from humans.	Blindness and skin disease	Tablets are taken annually and are donated by drug companies free of charge. Should demand exceed the donated amounts, drugs can be purchased for roughly $0.58.
Rabies	Unknown, though each year, more than 15 million people receive post-exposure drugs to prevent the onset of rabies.	Unknown	Worldwide	Domestic and wild animals	Bite of an infected animal.	In the early stages, fever and burning or itching at the wound site. As later stages, symptoms may include paralysis or hyperactivity. Rabies is always fatal if untreated.	Disinfection of the wound site and immunization. Post-exposure treatment costs between $40 and $50.

Appendix C. (Continued).

Disease	Prevalence (million)	Population at Risk (millions)	Regions of Highest Prevalence	Reservoir	Mode of Transmission	Symptoms	Treatment Availability and Cost
Schistosomiasis (bilharzia)	207	779	Sub-tropical areas of Asia; Latin America and Caribbean; and sub-Saharan Africa	Humans (primarily) and rodents	The egg of a parasitic flatworm is released in water through human urine or feces. Once the egg hatches, the larvae swim to find a mollusk host. There, the larvae develops into a cercariae, which enter the human body either through the skin or ingestion. In humans, cercariae mature and lay eggs that are discharged through urine or feces.	Urinary schistosomiasis damages the bladder, uterus and kidneys. Intestinal schistosomiasis causes enlargement of the liver and spleen, damages the intestines, and causes hypertension of the abdominal blood vessels.	Tablets are taken once or twice annually and are donated free of charge by drug manufacturers. Should demand exceed the donated amounts, drugs can be purchased for between \$0.32 and \$1.02 per person.
Soil-transmitted Helminths							
• Ascariasis (roundworm)	807	4,200	Tropical Areas	Humans	When humans carrying roundworm defecate on the ground, infective roundworm eggs in feces are deposited on the ground.	Malnutrition, stunting, and cognitive delays	Tablets are taken once or twice annually and are donated free of charge by drug manufacturers. Should demand exceed the

Appendix C. (Continued).

Disease	Prevalence (million)	Population at Risk (millions)	Regions of Highest Prevalence	Reservoir	Mode of Transmission	Symptoms	Treatment Availability and Cost
					Humans become infected when they eat produce grown in the contaminated soil or children eat the soil during or after play (poor handwashing). Ascariasis is not transmissible from person to person or from fresh feces. The worm eggs are infective when they are 2-3 weeks old, and may remain infective for several months or years in favorable soil. Mature female worms living in human intestines can produce more than 200,000 eggs daily.		

Appendix C. (Continued).

Disease	Prevalence (million)	Population at Risk (millions)	Regions of Highest Prevalence	Reservoir	Mode of Transmission	Symptoms	Treatment Availability and Cost
• Hookworm	576	3,200	Tropical and sub-tropical areas	Humans	When humans carrying hookworms defecate on the ground, eggs in feces are deposited on the ground. Within 7-10 days of hatching, the larvae become infective and can penetrate the skin (usually through the feet). Scientists have also documented transmission of hookworm larvae through breastmilk.	Anemia, malnutrition, poor pregnancy outcomes, growth and cognitive delays	donated amounts, drugs can be purchased for roughly $0.02 per tablet.
• Trichuriasis (whipworm)	604	3,200	Worldwide	Humans	Ingestion of larvae found in contaminated soil and on contaminated vegetables.	Inflammatory bowel disease, stunting, and cognitive delays	

Appendix C. (Continued).

Trachoma	84	590	Worldwide, primarily the Middle East; North and sub-Saharan Africa	Humans	Direct contact with infectious ocular or nasal discharges found on fingers and contaminated sources like towels, clothes. Flies also contribute to trachoma transmission.	Swelling and scarring of the eyelid. Trachoma can lead to blindness if left untreated.	According to WHO, pharmaceutical donations reportedly meet all needs as expressed by affected countries.
Treponematoses (yaws,bejel, and pinta)	Unknown	Unknown	Africa; Asia; Latin America	Humans and possibly higher primates	Direct contact with early skin lesions of infected people. Indirect transmission through contamination from scratching, skin-piercing articles and flies on open wounds Is probable, but of unknown importance.	Lesions, ulcers, and deterioration of facial tissues (nose and mouth) and bones.	Penicillin

Sources: Peter Hotez, Alan Fenwick, and Sonia Sachs, "Control of Neglected Tropical Diseases," *The New England Journal of Medicine*, vol. 357, no. 10 (September 6, 2007); pp. 1018-1027; *Control of Communicable Diseases Manual*, ed. David Heymann, 19th ed. (Washington, DC: APHA Press, 2008); *A Dictionary of Public Health*, ed. John Last (New York, NY: Oxford University Press, 2007); *A Dictionary of Epidemiology*, ed. Miquel Porta, 5th ed. (New York, NY: Oxford University Press, 2008), WHO, *First WHO Report on Neglected Tropical Diseases*, 2010; and E-mail from Project Manager, WHO Department of Control of Neglected Tropical Diseases, January 6, 2010.

Note: Three other NTDs are not included here because data on prevalence, morbidity, and mortality are limited. These are cysticercosis, echinococcosis, and foodborne trematode infections.

Appendix D. Images of Neglected Tropical Diseases

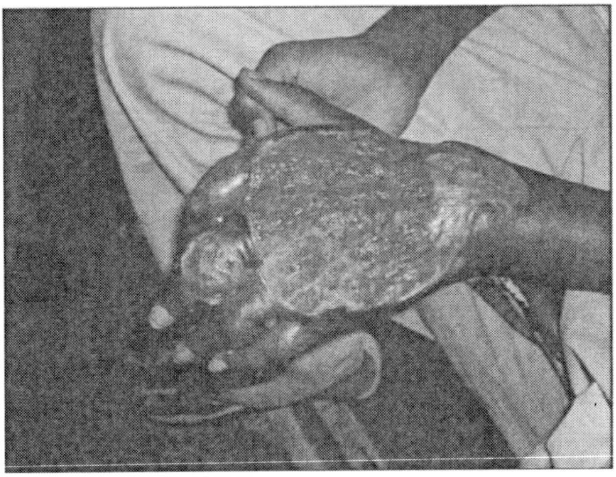

Source: http://www.cdc.gov/EID/content/13/5/782-G.htm.
Notes: A typical Buruli ulcer in a 17-year-old boy identified during the assessment.

Figure D-1. Buruli Ulcer.

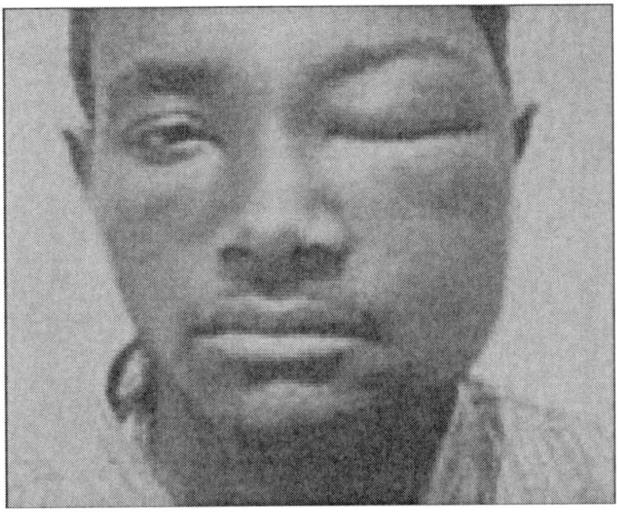

Source: http://iom.edu/~/media/Files/Activity%20Files/PublicHealth/MicrobialThreats/2010-SEP-21/Chang.pdf.

Figure D-2. Chagas.

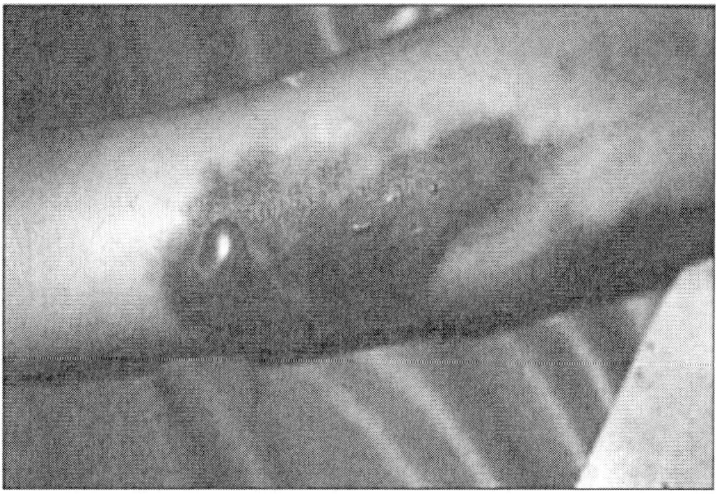

Source: http://www.topnews.in/health

Figure D-3. Dengue/dengue hemorrhagic fever.

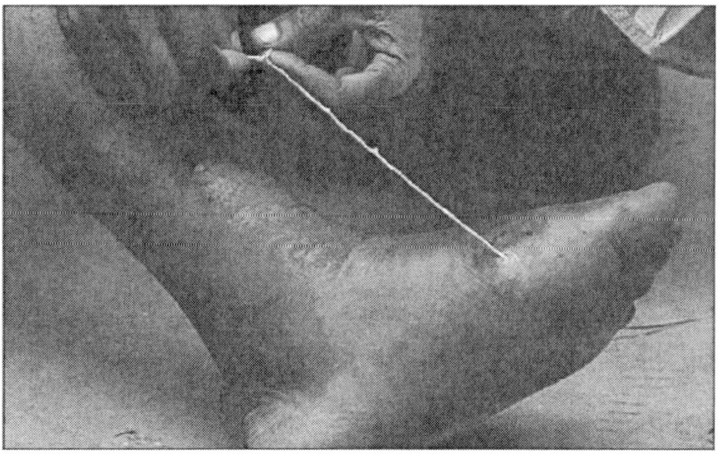

Source: http://graphics8.nytimes.com/images/2006/03/25/international/26worm_leg.jpg.

Figure D-4. Dracunculiasis (guinea-worm diseases).

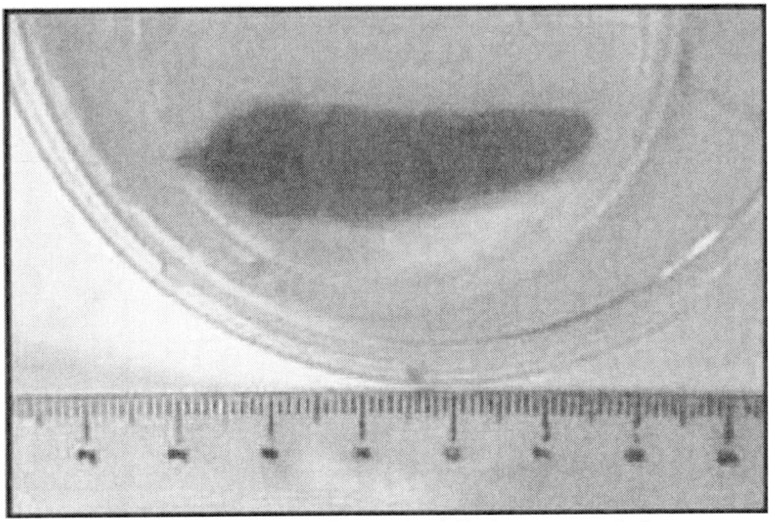

Source: http://www.who.int/neglected_diseasesFascioliasis_worm_ web. jpg.

Figure D-5. Fascioliasis.

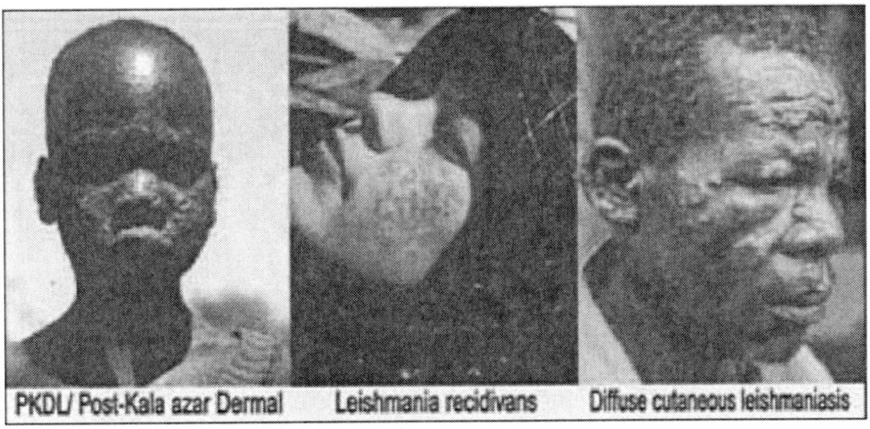

Source: http://www.who.int/leishmaniasis

Figure D-6. Leishmaniasis.

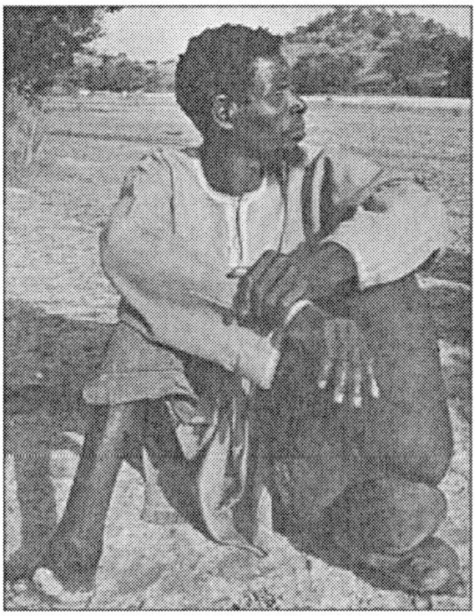

Source: http://www.nytimes.com/imagepages/2006/04/09/ world/09lymph_ CA1 ready.html.

Figure D-7. Lymphatic filariasis (elephantiasis).

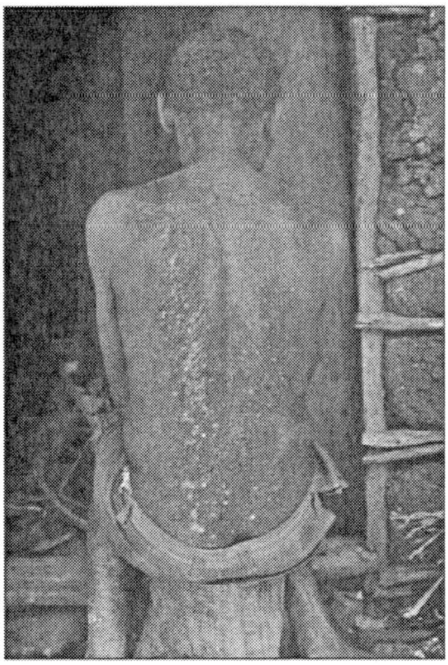

Source: http://www.neglecteddiseases.gov/newsroom/photo_galleries/ uganda/photo_ 03.html.

Figure D-8. Onchocerciasis (river blindness).

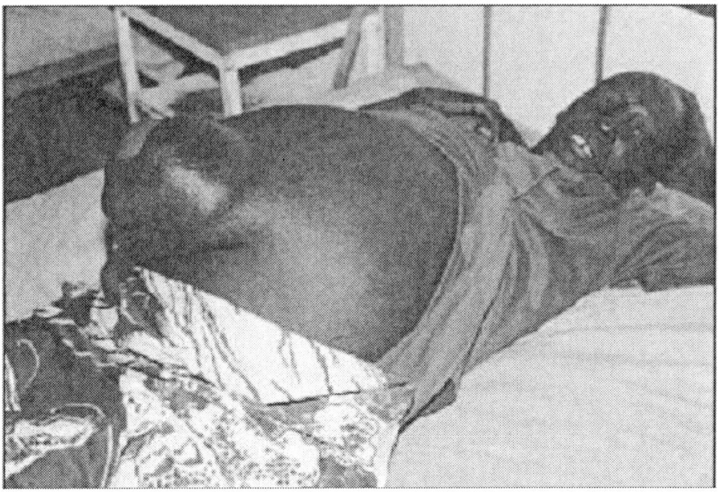

Source: http://www.abdn.ac.uk/ibes/research/int_phys/vector

Figure D-9. Schistosomiasis (bilharzia).

Soil-Trasmitted Helminthes

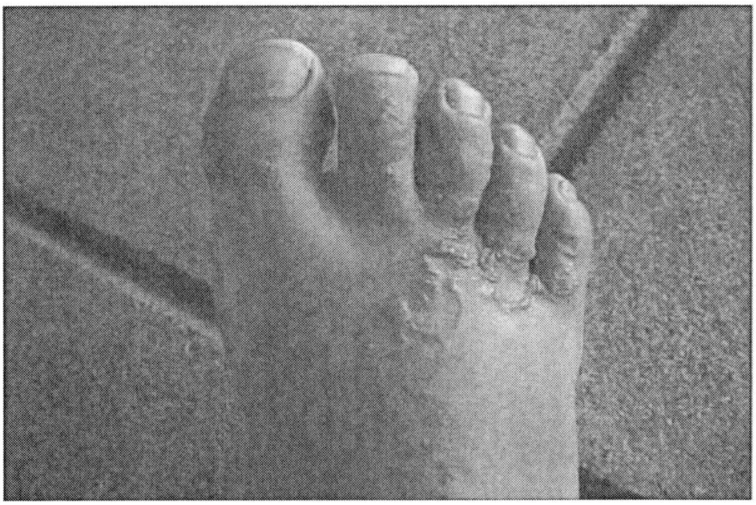

Source: http://scienceblogs.com/zooillogix/Hookworm%20Foot.jpg.

Figure D- 10. STH: Hookworm.

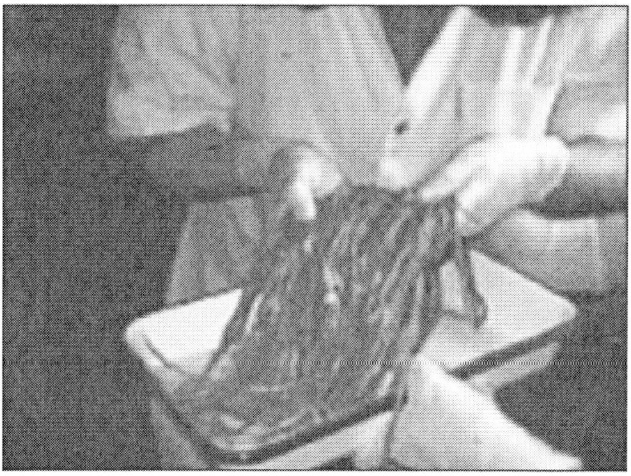

Source: http://neglecteddiseases.gov/target_diseases/soil_transmitted_ helminthiasis/roundworm/diagnosis.html.

Figure D-11. STH: Ascariasis (Roundworm).

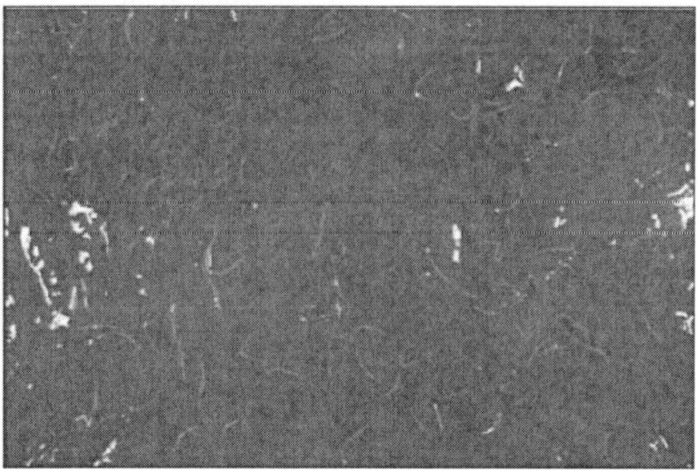

Source: http://www.stanford.edu/class/humbio103/ParaSites2002/trichuriasis.
Notes: Whipworm infection in the gut.

Figure D-12. STH: Trichuriasis (Whipworm).

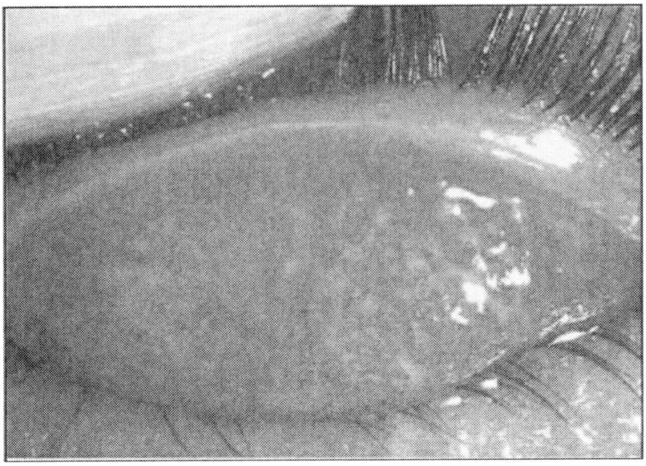

Source: http://www.who.int/blindness

Figure D-13. Trachoma.

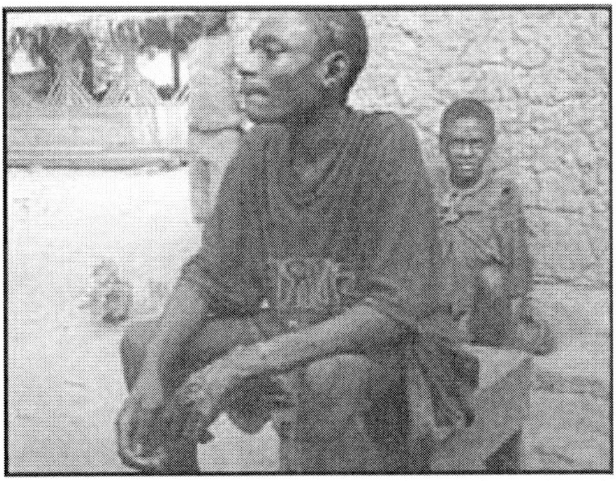

Source: http://www.who.int/mediacentre/factsheets/pian_033jaws_large.jp.
Notes: Man with Yaws in his left hand.

Figure D-14. Yaws.

Appendix E. Geographic Representation of NTD Co-Infection with HIV/AIDS, TB, and Malaria

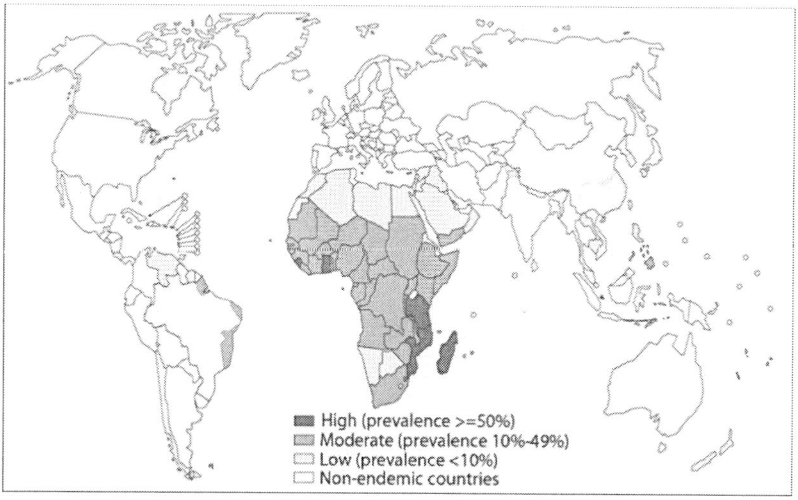

Source: WHO, Map Gallery at http://gamapserver.who.int/mapLibrary/Files/Maps/Global_schistosomiasis

Figure E-1. Global Distribution of Schistosomiasis, 2009.

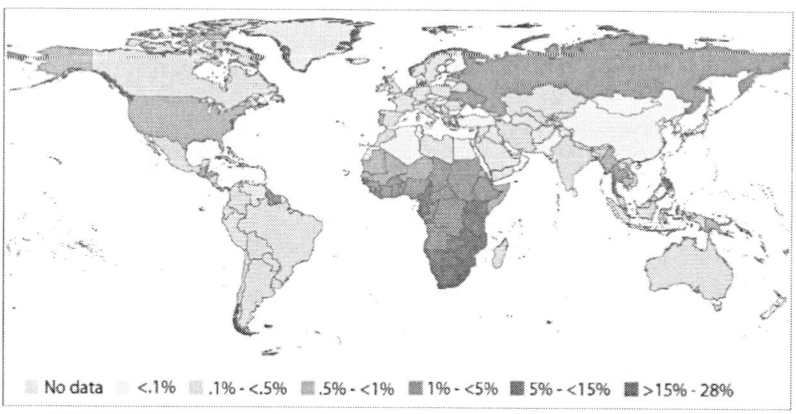

Source: UNAIDS, *Report on the Global AIDS Epidemic*, 2010, at http://www.unaids.org/globalreport/documents/ 20101123_globalreport_slides_chapter2_em.pdf.

Figure E-2. Global Prevalence of HIV/AIDS, 2009.

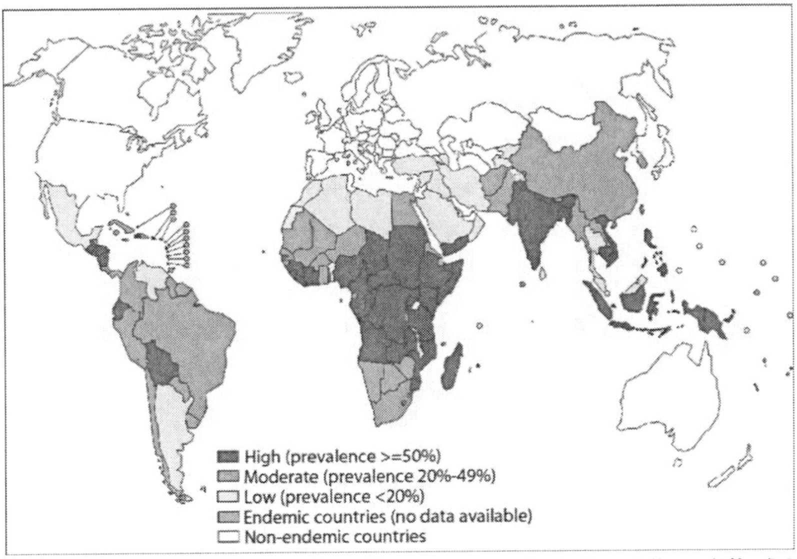

Source: WHO, Map Gallery at http://gamapserver.who.int/mapLibrary/Files/Maps/Global_STH_2009.png.

Figure E-3. Global Distribution of Soil-Transmitted Helminths, 2009.

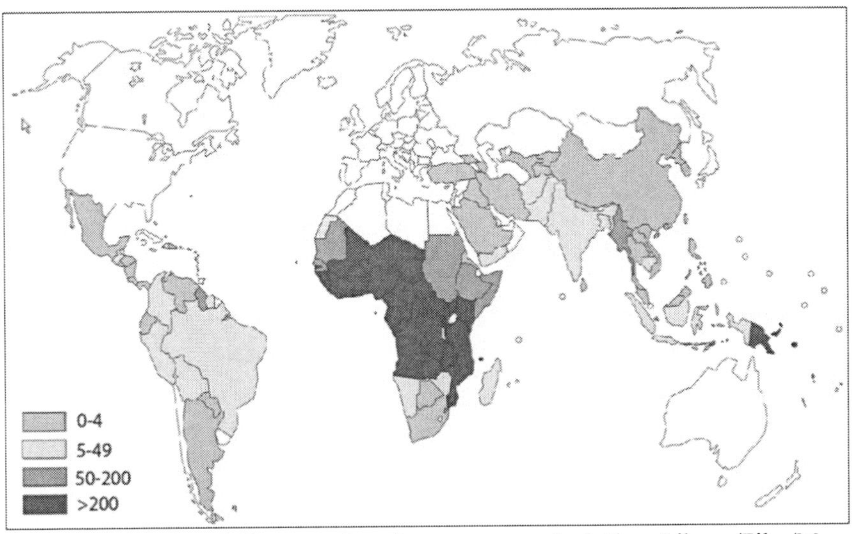

Source: WHO, Map Gallery at http://gamapserver.who.int/mapLibrary/Files/Maps/Malaria_Incidence_2006.png.

Figure E-4. Estimated Global Incidence of Malaria, 2006.

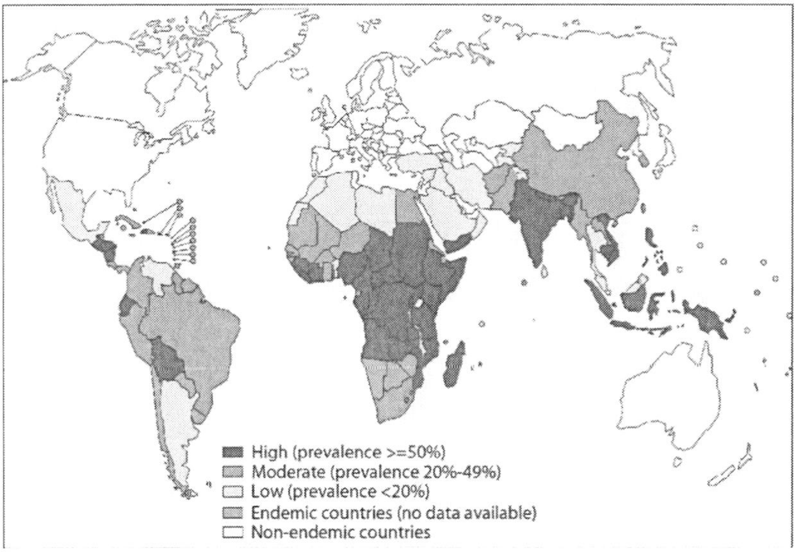

Source: WHO, Map Gallery at http://gamapserver.who.int/mapLibrary/Files/Maps/Global_STH_2009.png.

Figure E-5. Global Distribution of Soil-Transmitted Helminths, 2009.

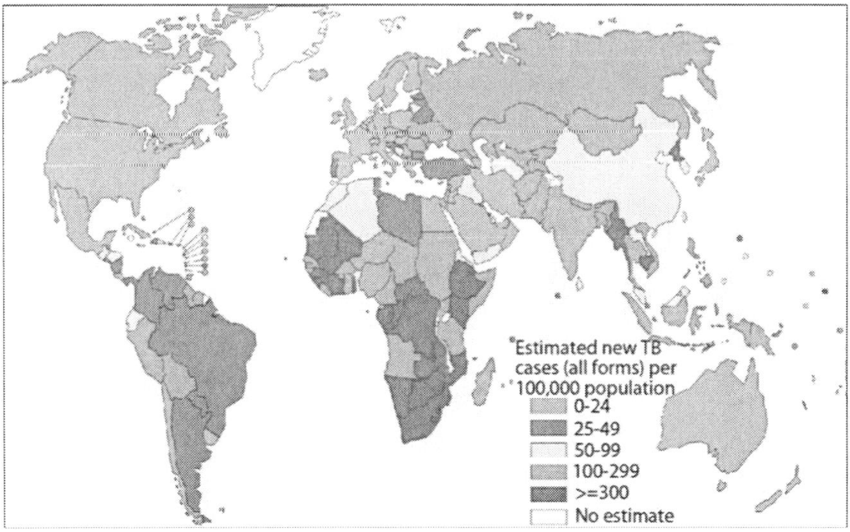

Source: WHO, Map Gallery at http://gamapserver.who.int/mapLibrary/Files/Maps/TBincidence_2009.png.

Figure E-6. Estimated Global TB Incidence Rates, 2009.

Appendix F. Key Initiatives to Fight NTDs

Multi-Disease Initiatives		
Organizations	Goal	Diseases Covered
World Health Organization[103]	• Eliminate or eradicate NTDs targeted in resolutions of the World Health Assembly and regional committees; • Reduce the burden of other tool-ready diseases; and • Ensure that interventions using novel approaches are available, promoted and accessible for tool-deficient diseases. • cysticercosis, dracunculiasis (guinea-worm disease), echinococcosis, foodborne trematode infections, lymphatic filariasis, onchocerciasis (river blindness) schistosomiasis (bilharziasis) and soil transmitted helminthiasis.	Buruli Ulcer Chagas disease (American trypanosomiasis) Dengue/dengue haemorrhagic fever Dracunculiasis (guinea-worm disease) Fascioliasis Human African trypanosomiasis Leishmaniasis Leprosy Lymphatic filariasis Onchocerciasis Rabies Schistosomiasis Soil transmitted helminthiasis (ascariasis, hookworm, and trichuriasis) Snakebite Trachoma Yaws
Global Network for Neglected Tropical Diseases[104]	Raise the awareness, political will, and funding necessary to control and eliminate the seven most common NTDs	Lymphatic filariasis Onchocerciasis Schistosomiasis Soil-transmitted helminths Trachoma

Appendix F. (Continued).

Multi-Disease Initiatives		
Organizations	Goal	Diseases Covered
The U.S. Neglected Tropical Disease Program [105]	• Supply 1 billion NTD treatments; • Halve the prevalence of seven NTDs in 30 countries by 2013 that account for 70% of the global disease burden of the targeted diseases; • Eliminate onchocerciasis in Latin America by 2016; • Eliminate leprosy in all endemic countries by 2016; and • Eliminate lymphatic filariasis globally by 2020.	Lymphatic filariasis Onchocerciasis Schistosomiasis Soil-transmitted helminths Trachoma
Single-Disease Initiative		
Initiatives for the Seven Most Common NTDs	Goal	Partners
Global Alliance to Eliminate Lymphatic Filiariasis[106]	Eliminate globally as a public health problem by 1997	More than forty partners from the public and private sectors, academia, international development organizations and NGOs
Onchocerciasis Control Program (OCP), African Program for Onchocerciasis Control (APOC), and Onchocerciasis Elimination Program for the Americas (OEPA)[107]	Eliminate regionally by 2008 (APOC): 1995-2015, 65% coverage with MDA	Fifteen partners including NGOs, the World Bank, and pharmaceutical companies
Shistosomiasis Control Initiative[108]	Reduce disease through periodic, targeted treatment with praziquantel	Sixteen partners including academia, international development organizations, NGOs and national governments

Appendix F. (Continued).

Multi-Disease Initiatives		
Organizations	Goal	Diseases Covered
The Partnership for Parasite Control[109]	Regularly treat at least 75% of all school-aged children at risk of illness from schistosomiasis and soil transmitted helminths by 2010	PPC is composed of various UN agencies, research institutes, universities and a multitude of NGOs who work together to reduce illness and death caused by schistosomiasis and soil-transmitted helminithes
Global Elimination of Trachoma by 2020 (GET 2020)[110] and International Trachoma Initiative[111]	Eliminate by 2020; eliminate "blinding trachoma" by 1998	A partnership between WHO, Member States, NGOs, foundations, and the private sector
Other NTD Initiatives	Goal	Partners
Elimination of Chagas [112]	Eliminate disease transmission by 1998; control and elimination by 2010	PAHO
Elimination of leprosy[113]	Eliminate as a global health problem, 1991; Eliminate as a public health problem, 1998. Ensure accessible, uninterrupted, sustainable MDA	National programs in those countries endemic with the disease; World Bank, UNICEF, UNHCR and UNDP
Elimination of visceral leishmaniasis[114]	Eliminate regionally by 2015	Ministers of Health of Bangladesh, India and Nepal, WHO/PAHO
Guinea Worm Eradication Program	Eradicate globally by 2004	CDC, The Carter Center, DFID, WHO, the United Nations Children's Fund and the Bill & Melinda Gates Foundation

Appendix F. (Continued).

Multi-Disease Initiatives		
Organizations	Goal	Diseases Covered
Program to Eliminate Sleeping Sickness	• Strengthen and coordinate control measures • Strengthen surveillance system • Monitor treatment and drug resistance • Develop information database and training activities	Aventis Pharma (now Sanofi-aventis), Bayer, other private partners, NGOs, and Belgian and French bilateral cooperation projects

APPENDIX G. OTHER NTD PROGRAMS

Over the past two decades, several groups have sought to increase the availability and access to treatment for NTDs in high-burdened countries. These outfits are diverse in their mission; some were established to provide treatment for a specific NTD, such as onchocerciasis, while others are regional elimination efforts. A majority of these partnerships focus on the procurement and supply of drugs, while some incorporate advocacy functions and others focus on R&D for new drugs. Below are prominent examples of groups that offer NTD programs. This list is not exhaustive.

Bill & Melinda Gates Foundation[115]

The Gates Foundation targets a specific set of NTDs, including cysticercosis, dengue, guinea-worm disease, soil-transmitted helminths, Human African trypanosomiasis, Human papillomavirus, Japanese encephalitis, lymphatic filariasis, onchocerciasis, schistosomiasis, trachoma, and lesishmaniasis.[116] Between 1998 and 2009, the Gates Foundation provided more than $717 million for 163 NTD projects and contributions to international organizations and public-private partnerships, including WHO, the Guinea Worm Eradication Program and the Global Network for Neglected Tropical Diseases.

Carter Center[117]

The Carter Center the Center focuses on six diseases: dracunculiasis (guinea worm), onchocerciasis (river blindness), trachoma, schistosomiasis, lymphatic filariasis, and malaria. The Carter Center is possible best known for its leading role in eliminating guinea worm. Efforts launched in 1986 by the Carter Center have contributed to a 99% reduction in global incidence of guinea worm. In 1997, the Carter Center expanded its focus on diseases to include health system strengthening.

Children without Worms[118]

Children Without Worms is a partnership between Johnson & Johnson and The Task Force for Global Health (formerly the Task Force for Child Survival and Development) working to reduce the burden of soil-transmitted helminth infections in children from eight countries in Latin America, Africa, and Asia. Children Without Worms uses annual donations of medendazole from Johnson & Johnson and targets its distribution based on the size and need of local populations.

Drugs for Neglected Diseases Initiative (DNDi)[119]

In 2003, seven organizations launched DNDi to work in partnership with the pharmaceutical industry, academia and non-governmental organizations to develop new treatments for NTDs and strengthen research capacity in African and Asian countries. DNDi focuses on the development of new drugs for the most neglected diseases, such as Human African trypanosomiasis (sleeping sickness), visceral leishmaniasis, and Chagas disease. The primary objective of DNDi is the delivery of six to eight new treatments for leishmaniasis, Human African trypanosomiasis, Chagas disease, and malaria by 2014.

Global Network for Neglected Tropical Diseases[120]

The Global Network for Neglected Tropical Disease is a partnership launched in September 2006 to advocate for controlling and reducing the burden of NTDs. This partnership seeks to raise the profile of NTDs as a global health issue through advocacy, resource mobilization and global coordination efforts. Communicating success stories is an important component of the Network's work, through sharing personal stories, highlighting disease-specific achievements, and communicating progress in the field.

International Vaccine Institute[121]

The International Vaccine Initiative (IVI) is an international center of research, training, and technical assistance that aims to develop vaccines against diseases that plague developing countries. As of October 2010, 33 countries became signatories and an additional 16 countries were party to the initiative. The United States is not a signatory or party to the South Korean-based initiative, though WRAIR and CDC partners with IVI in various capacities (e.g., researching a vaccine against dengue) and the Bill & Melinda Gates Foundation serves as a key donor. IVI scientists have developed a vaccine against cholera and an IVI-developed vaccine against typhoid fever was 80% effective during a phase 4 trial.[122]

Infectious Diseases Research Institute[123]

The Infectious Diseases Research Institute (IDRI) is a Seattle-based non-profit research center aimed at applying innovative science to the research and development of products to prevent, detect and treat infectious diseases of poverty. IDRI is currently researching treatments against leishmaniasis, TB, malaria, leprosy, and Chagas.

Institute for One World Health[124]

The Institute for One World Health is a non-profit organization aimed at developing safe, effective, and affordable new medicines to treat infectious diseases that are commonly found in poorer countries. The institute is currently focusing on developing new treatments against leishmaniasis, diarrheal diseases, malaria, Chagas, and soil-transmitted diseases.

Pharmaceutical Industry

Primarily through large donations of NTD treatments for little or no cost, the pharmaceutical industry plays an important role in global NTD initiatives. Key pharmaceutical companies include Bayer HealthCare, GlaxoSmithKline, Johnson & Johnson, MedPharm, Merck Inc., Merck KGaA, Novartis, Pfizer, and Sanofi-aventis. One example of the pharmaceutical industry's central role to the global response to NTDs is Merck's Mectizan Donation Program. Launched in 1987, the effort stands as the longest-running disease-specific drug donation program. Merck initiated the initiative with large quantities of free Mectizan to treat onchocerciasis and expanded the program in 1998 to target lymphatic filariasis. In a 2008 report, Merck indicated that it had donated more than 2.5 billion tablets of Mectizan that were used to treat 80 million people in Latin America, Africa, and the Middle East.[125]

Sabin Vaccine Institute[126]

The Sabine Vaccine Institute is a non-profit organization that advocates for and engages in R&D of innovative vaccines to prevent the spread of infectious and neglected tropical diseases. The institute is currently focusing on developing vaccines against hookworm, schistosomiasis, and malaria. The Sabin Institute also supports technology transfer to less developed countries, such as efforts with Brazil.

Special Program for Research and Training in Tropical Diseases[127]

The Special Program for Research and Training in Tropical Diseases (TDR) was established in 1975 to support the development of new tools to fight tropical diseases and strengthen the research capacity of affected developing countries. The program is executed by WHO and cosponsored by UNDP, the United Nations Children's Fund (UNICEF), and the World Bank. TDR anticipates facilitating the elimination of four NTDS globally: Chagas disease, leprosy, lymphatic filariasis, and onchocerciasis. It also aims to eliminate visceral leishmaniasis in Latin America. According to the TDR Business Plan for 2008-2013, none of the targeted diseases can be eradicated with current tools and investments, though regional elimination can be achieved.[128]

Donor contributions to TDR have increased over the past decade from $57 million in the 2000- 2001 budget period to $77.5 million between 2008 and 2009. The United States is a key donor to TDR, though U.S. contributions have declined over the past decade. During 2000-2001, the U.S. contributed $9.2 million, or 16% of total contributions.[129] Between 2008 and 2009 U.S. contributions totaled $4.8 million, amounting to roughly 6% of all contributions.[130]

ACKNOWLEDGMENTS

Craig Moscetti, former CRS analyst in Global Health, contributed to this report.

End Notes

[1] Appendix A lists acronyms, and Appendix B defines health terms that are used throughout the report.

[2] WHO, "The evidence is in: deworming helps meet the Millennium Development Goals," 2005.

[3] For more information on this meeting, see WHO, *Intensified Control of Neglected Diseases*, Report of an International Workshop, December 2003.

[4] WHO, *Strategic and Technical Meeting on Intensified Control of Neglected Tropical Diseases*, Report of an International Workshop, 2006.

[5] WHO, *A Turning Point 2007: Report of the Global Partners' Meeting on Neglected Tropical Diseases*, Geneva, Switzerland, April 2007, p. ii; and Kaiser Family Foundation, *U.S. Global Health Policy Fact Sheet: Neglected Tropical Diseases*, July 2009. WHO, *Neglected Tropical Diseases: Hidden Success, Emerging Opportunities*, 2009.

[6] Philip Musgrove and Peter Hotez, "Turning Neglected Tropical Diseases Into Forgotten Maladies," *Health Affairs*, vol. 28, no. 6 (November/December 2009), p. 1695.

[7] Dr. Margaret Chan, Director-General, *Address to the WHO Global Partners Meeting on Neglected Tropical Diseases*, WHO, April 19, 2007.

[8] For a list of World Health Assembly resolutions related to tackling NTDs, see WHO, *First WHO Report on Neglected Tropical Diseases*, 2010.

[9] WHO, *Integrated Control of the Neglected Tropical Diseases: A Neglected Opportunity Ripe for Action*, May 2008, p. 3.

[10] Countries terminate mass drug administration (MDA) campaigns after the disease no longer causes a significant disease burden. After ending an MDA campaign, WHO conducts research to confirm no new cases have occurred for at least three years. After this period, WHO classifies the disease as eliminated. Disease surveillance must be sustained, because the agent causing the disease is still present and can cause a resurgence of illness. Eradication, in contrast, means the agent causing the disease is no longer present and does not threaten human health.

[11] Personal communication with USAID, Infectious Diseases Division, November 5, 2010.

[12] WHO, *Global Plan to Combat Neglected Tropical Diseases 2008-2015*, 2007.

[13] WHO, *First WHO Report on Neglected Tropical Diseases*, 2010.

[14] See Donald Hopkins and P. Craig Withers, *Sudan's War and Eradication of Dracunculiasis*, Carter Center, March 18, 2003.

[15] PAHO and WHO, *Elimination of Neglected Diseases and Other Poverty-Related Infections*, July 10, 2009, p. 3.

[16] Merck & Co., "Public Health Officials Announce First Country to Eliminate Transmission of the Tropical Disease Onchocerciasis," press release, November 15, 2007.

[17] WHO, *First WHO Report on Neglected Tropical Diseases*, 2010, p. 124 and Julie Jacobson, "Neglected & Other Infectious Diseases: Bill & Melinda Gates Foundation," Presentation at the Institute of Medicine conference on NTDs, Washington, DC, September 23, 2010, p. 14.

[18] Section 593, P.L. 109-102, FY2006 Foreign Operations Appropriations.

[19] The seven NTDs are lymphatic filariasis (elephantiasis); schistosomiasis (snail fever); trachoma (eye infection); onchocerciasis (river blindness); and three soil-transmitted helminths (STHs—hookworm, roundworm, whipworm). See White House, "President Bush Announces New Global Initiative To Combat Neglected Tropical Diseases," press release, February 20, 2008.

[20] USAID, HHS, CDC & Department of State, *Lantos-Hyde United States Government Malaria Strategy, 2009-2014*, April 2010.

[21] Department of State, *Implementation of the Global Health Initiative: Consultation Document*, February 2010, p. 20.

[22] Personal communication with USAID, Infectious Disease Division, USAID, December 27, 2010.

[23] Ibid. At the time this report was published, only 12 countries were listed on the NTD Program website.

[24] Information in this section was drawn from personal communication with USAID, Infectious Disease Division, December 10, 2010.

[25] CDC, National Center for Zoonotic, Vector-Borne and Enteric Diseases, "Parasitic Diseases Brach," August 2009.

[26] NIH, "NIH Announces New Program to Develop Therapeutics for Rare and Neglected Diseases," press release, May 20, 2009.

[27] NIAID webpage on its role in NTD research at http://www.niaid.nih.gov/topics/tropical Diseases/research/Pages/ role.aspx, accessed on November 20, 2010.

[28] Unless otherwise indicated, information in this section is drawn from U.S. Army Medical Research and Materiel Command, *USAMRMC Product Portfolio*, June 2007.

[29] These facilities include the Global Emerging Infections System, the Walter Reed Army Institute of Research, Naval Medical Research Centers, and regional commands, including U.S. Africa Command. For more information on DOD's foreign assistance, see CRS Report RL34639, *The Department of Defense Role in Foreign Assistance: Background, Major Issues, and Options for Congress*, coordinated by Nina M. Serafino.

[30] USAID, *The Modern Development Enterprise*, Remarks by Dr. Rajiv Shah at the Center for Global Development, January 19, 2011.

[31] Eran Bendavid et al., "The Relation of Price of Antiretroviral Drugs and Foreign Assistance with Coverage of HIV Treatment in Africa: Retrospective Study," *British Medical Journal*, vol. 341 (November 18, 2010), p. c6218.

[32] Members of the Malaria and NTD Caucus, *Letter to USAID Administrator Rajiv Shah*, March 23, 2010.

[33] After detecting the parasite that causes Chagas disease in the U.S. blood supply, the U.S. Food and Drug Administration (FDA) required in May 2004 that all blood donated throughout the United States be tested for Chagas. FDA, *Draft Guidance for Industry: Use of Serological Tests to Reduce the Risk of Transmission of Trypanosoma cruzi Infection in Whole Blood and Blood Components for Transfusion and Human Cells, Tissues, and Cellular and Tissue-Based Products*, March 2009.

[34] See Section 593, P.L. 109-102, FY2006 Foreign Operations Appropriations.

[35] PAHO and WHO, *Elimination of Neglected Diseases and Other Poverty-Related Infections*, July 10, 2009, p. 3.

[36] Merck & Co., "Public Health Officials Announce First Country to Eliminate Transmission of the Tropical Disease Onchocerciasis," press release, November 15, 2007.

[37] See Burton Singer, "Viewpoint by Burton Singer: Bring Back Primary Prevention for Relieving the Burden of NTDs," *PLoS Medicine*, vol. 7, no. 5 (May 2010), p. e1000255; and TR Burkot et al., "The Argument for Integrating Vector Control with Multiple Drug Administration Campaigns to Ensure Elimination of Lymphatic Filiariasis," *Filaria Journal*, vol. 5, no. 10 (August 2006).

[38] See, P J Hotez, "Mass Drug Administration and Integrated Control for the World's High-Prevalence Neglected Tropical Diseases," *Clinical Pharmacology & Therapeutics*, vol. 85, no. 6 (June 2009), pp. 659-664.

[39] Archie Clements et al., "A Comparative Study of the Spatial Distribution of Schistosomiasis in Mali in 1984-1989 and 2004-2006," *PLoS Neglected Tropical Diseases*, vol. 3, no. 5 (May 2009), p. e431.

[40] Anna Cavalli et al., "Interactions between Global Health Initiatives and Country Health Systems: The Case of a Neglected Tropical Diseases Control Program in Mali," *PLoS Neglected Tropical Diseses*, vol. 4, no. 8 (August 2010), p. e798.

[41] In June 2010, the Center for Global Development (CGD) recorded an event where key stakeholders debated how to enhance country ownership of health programs. See http://blogs.

[42] See Margaret Chan et al., "Meeting the Demand for Results and Accountability: A Call for Action on Health Data from Eight Global Health Agencies," *PLoS Medicine*, vol. 7, no. 1 (January 26, 2010), p. e1000223; and Lawrence O. Gostin and Emily A. Mok, "Grand Challenges in Global Health Governance," *British Medical Bulletin*, vol. 90, no. 1 (April 17, 2009), pp. 7-18.

[43] Gavin Yamey, "The Unsung Hero of Neglected Tropical Diseases: Interview with Narcis Kabatereine," *PLoS Neglected Tropical Diseases*, vol. 3, no. 12 (December 2009), p. e546.

[44] Mary Linehan et al., "Integrated Implemenation of Programs Targeting Neglected Tropical Diseases Through Preventive Chemotherapy: Proving the Feasiblity at National-Scale," *American Journal of Tropical Medicine and Hygiene*, vol. 84, no. 1 (2011), pp. 5-14.

[45] For more information on GHI, see http://www.pepfar.gov/ghi/index.htm.

[46] John Donnelly, *Shah: 'We Want Real Outcomes Health'*, Aspen Global Health and Development, September 15, 2010, http://www.ministerial-leadership

[47] See the PEPFAR website on Partnership Frameworks at http://www.pepfar.gov/frameworks/.

[48] Ambassador Eric Goosby advocated the application of the Partnership Framework in his statement for U.S. Congress, House Committee on Foreign Affairs, *PEPFAR: From Emergency to Sustainability and Advances Against HIV/AIDS*, 111th Cong., September 29, 2010, see http://internationalrelations.house.gov/111/goo092910.pdf.

[49] Personal communication with USAID, Infectious Diseases Division, November 5, 2010.

[50] See the webpage for the "15 by 2015" campaign at http://www.15by2015.org/.

[51] Louis Lambrechts et al., "Shifting Priorities in Vector Biology to Improve Control of Vector-Borne Disease," *Tropical Medicine and International* Health, vol. 14, no. 12 (December 2009).

[52] Marcia C. Castro et al., "The Importance of Drains for the Larval Development of Lymphatic Filariasis and Malaria Vectors in Dar es Salaam, United Republic of Tanzania," *PLoS Neglected Tropical Diseases*, vol. 4, no. 5 (May 2010).

[53] L. Chitsulo et al., "The global status of schistosomiasis and its control," *Acta Tropica*, vol. 77, no. 1 (October 23, 2000), pp. 41-51.

[54] For examples of the role of vector control in eradicating NTDs, see Darren J Gray et al., "Schistosomiasis Elimination: Lessons From the Past Guide the Future," *The Lancet*, vol. 10, no. 10 (October 2010), pp. 733-736; and Moses J. Bockarie et al., "Role of Vector

Control in the Global Program to Eliminate Lymphatic Filariasis," *The Annual Review of Entomology*, vol. 54 (January 2009), pp. 469-487.

[55] In the early 1900s, the Rockefeller Foundation and its implementing partners combined wide-scale sanitation projects with drug administration and public education to eliminate hookworm infections, which plagued much of the southeastern United States at the time. For more on this approach, see E.A. Alderman et al., *The Rockefeller Sanitary Commission for the Eradication of Hookworm Disease* (Washington, DC: Offices of the Commission, 1915). This book is available on-line at http://www.archive.org/details/cu31924005710839.

[56] See CDC, *WASH Away Neglected Tropical Diseases*, Activity Summary, June 2010, http://www.cdc.gov/ healthywater/pdf/global/programs/wash-away-ntd-summary.pdf and CDC, *WASH Away Neglected Tropical Diseases*, Program in Brief, June 2010.

[57] Philip Musgrove and Peter Hotez, "Turning Neglected Tropical Diseases Into Forgotten Maladies," *Health Affairs*, vol. 28, no. 6 (November/December 2009), p. 1698.

[58] Charles H King, "Toward the Elimination of Schistosomiasis," *New England Journal of Medicine*, vol. 360, no. 2 (October 29, 2010), pp. 106-109.

[59] Tan Ee Lyn, *China to Help Africa to Curb Chronic Snail Fever*, Reuters, October 6, 2010.

[60] Jennifer Keiser et al., "Effect of irrigated rice agriculture on Japanese encephalitis, including challenges and opportunities for integrated vector management," *Acta Tropica* , vol. 95, no. 1 (July 2005), pp. 40-57.

[61] Sung-Tae Hong et al., "A Successful Experience of Soil-Transmitted Helminth Control in the Republic of Korea," *Korean Journal of Parasitology*, vol. 44, no. 3 (September 2006), pp. 177-185.

[62] Ricardo E. Gürtler et al., "Sustainable vector control and management of Chagas disease in the Gran Chaco, Argentina," *PNAS*, vol. 104, no. 41 (October 9, 2007), p. 16194-16199.

[63] USAID, *Neglected Tropical Disease Control Program*, Semi Annual Report, November 1, 2009, p. 16.

[64] Peter Hotez et al., "Incorporating a Rapid-Impact Package for Neglected Tropical Diseases with Programs for HIV/AIDS, Tuberculosis, and Malaria," *PLoS Medicine*, vol. 3, no. 5 (May 2006), pp. 576-584.

[65] The concept of integrative NTD projects is explored extensively in Burton H. Singer and Marcia Caldas de Castro, "Bridges to sustainable tropical health," *PNAS*, vol. 104, no. 41 (October 9, 2007), p. 16038–16043.

[66] See U.S. Department of State, *Senator Paul Simon Water for the Poor Act: Report to Congress*, June 2010.

[67] Hillary Rodham Clinton, *The Global Health Initiative: The Next Phase of American Leadership*, Secretary of State, Speech at the Johns Hopkins School of Advanced International Studies, August 16, 2010.

[68] Personal communication with USAID, Infectious Diseases Division, December 23, 2010.

[69] For more information on MCC and CDC water and sanitation programs, see http://www.mcc.gov/pages/activities/activity/water-and-sanitation and http://www.cdc.gov/safewater/about_pages/about_where.htm, respectively.

[70] For example, research could help to discover possible complications when undergoing NTD treatments while using traditional medicines. WHO estimates that 80% of African patients also use traditional medicines. See David J. Winters, "Expanding Global Research and Development for Neglected Diseases," *Bulletin of the World Health Organization*, vol. 84, no. 5 (May 2006), p. 414.

[71] Peter Hotez et al., "Incorporating a Rapid-Impact Package for Neglected Tropical Diseases with Programs for HIV/AIDS, Tuberculosis, and Malaria," *PLoS Medicine*, vol. 3, no. 5 (May 2006), pp. 576-584.

[72] M C Thomson et al., "Satellite Mapping of Loa Loa Prevalence in Relation to Ivermectin Use in West and Central Africa," *The Lancet*, vol. 356, no. 9235 (September 23, 2000), pp. 1077-1078. Although USAID only supports the administration of drugs for the seven most common NTDs and does not offer treatments for diseases like sleeping sickness and lesihmaniasis, it reportedly supports efforts to monitor severe adverse reactions against several NTD drugs, including sleeping sickness and leishmaniasis. Personal communication with USAID, Infectious Diseases Division, December 23, 2010.

[73] Participants of a June 2009 DNDi regional workshop on MRA, reportedly indicated that weak regulatory capacity in developing countries complicated efforts to expand access to NTD drugs. Dr Mary Moran et al., *Registering New Drugs: The African Context*, The George Institute for International Health and DNDi, January 2010, p. 2. A study conducted by WHO in 2006 found that over 40 African MRAs were insufficiently functional and needed significant capacity building to perform fundamental regulatory tasks. South Africa was the only country in sub-Saharan Africa with a fully functional MRA; the MRAs of Nigeria, Zimbabwe, Senegal, Tunisia, Morocco and Algeria were functional but needed "strengthening in regulation of clinical trials" among other things; and the MRAs of Ghana, Egypt, Uganda and Ethiopia had "potential" but were not yet fully functional. In 2005, 87% of African MRAs reported that they could not evaluate biologics such as vaccines, while some African MRAs did not yet have a vaccine registration system. Ibid., p. 6.

[74] WHO, *Country Pharmaceutical Situations*, Fact Book on WHO Level 1 indicators 2007, April 2009, p. 36, http://www.who.int/medicines/publications/EMP_MPC_2010_1.pdf.

[75] As discussed earlier (see "Defining "NTDs"), there are varying accounts of which diseases are considered NTDs. While conducting a study on global funding for NTD-related R&D, for example, a research organization called the George Institute for International Health counted HIV/AIDS, TB, and malaria among NTDs. While some groups consider these three diseases to be NTDs, CRS follows the WHO classification system and does not include HIV/AIDS, TB, or malaria among NTDs. The report remains useful, however, because it offers an analysis of R&D funding for several diseases including NTDs, which is not widely available.

[76] Members of the Malaria and NTD Caucus, *Letter to USAID Administrator Rajiv Shah*, March 23, 2010, http://www.dndi.org/images/stories/pdf_events/NTD%20Letter%20from%20Congress_March2010.pdf.

[77] Sec. 740, P.L. 111-80.

[78] In September 2010, the Neglected Disease Group held hosted a public hearing to discuss how the FDA could improve its global health work. The group is expected to report its recommendations to Congress in March 2011. See FDA, "Advancing the Development of Medical Products Used in the Prevention, Diagnosis, and Treatment of Neglected Tropical Diseases; Public Hearing," 75 *Federal Register* 42103, July 20, 2010.

[79] See FDA, *The FDA's Role in Global Health*, Fact Sheet, September 2010, p. 2.

[80] Tom Bollyky, *Right Hearing, Wrong Message on Neglected Pediatric Diseases*, Center for Global Development, Global Health Policy Blog, July 29, 2010, http://blogs. nl_weekly_08182010.

[81] See Stefano Villa, Amelia Compagni, and Michael R. Reich, "Orphan Drug Legislation: Lessons for Neglected Tropical Diseases," *International Journal of Health Planning and Management*, vol. 24, no. 1 (April 24, 2008), pp. 27-42.

[82] See Sarah E. Frew, Victor Y. Liu, and Peter A. Singer, "A Business Plan To Help The 'Global South' In Its Fight Against Neglected Diseases," *Health Affairs*, vol. 28, no. 6 (November/December 2009), pp. 1760-1773; and Mary Moran, "A Breakthrough in R&D for Neglected Tropical Diseasses: New Ways to Get the Drugs We Need," *PLoS Medicine*, vol. 2, no. 9 (September 2005), pp. 828-832.

[83] See the TDR website at http://apps.who.int/tdr/ and the DND*i* website at http://www.dndi.org/.

[84] WHO and TDR, *Innovation for Health: Research That Makes a Difference*, 2009 Annual Report, p. 70.

[85] DND*i*, *Delivering Innovation and Building a Robust Pipeline*, 2008-20009 Annual Report, p. 57.

[86] Philip Hosbach and Stuart Feldman, "Dengue Fever—An Escalating Threat," *Global Health* , Fall 2010.

[87] CDC, "Locally Acquired Dengue: Key West, Florida 2009-2010," *Morbidity and Mortality Weekly Report*, vol. 59, no. 19 (May 21, 2010), pp. 577-581.

[88] Crystal Franco et al., *Biosecurity and Bioterrorism: Biodefense Strategy, Practice, and Science*, vol. 8, no. 3 (2010).

[89] For a complete list of "Nationally Notifiable Diseases," see http://www.cdc.gov/ncphi/disss/nndss/phs/ infdis2010.htm.

[90] F J Carod-Artal et al., "American Trypanosomiasis (Chagas' Disease): An Unrecognised Cause of Stroke," *Journal of Neurology, Neurosurgery, and Psychiatry*, vol. 74 (2003), pp. 516-518.

[91] WHO, *Schistosomiasis*, Fact Sheet, February 2010.

[92] H.R. 5986, Neglected Infections of Impoverished Americans Act of 2010.

[93] Chris Beyrer, "Neglected Diseases, Civil Conflicts,and the Right to Health," Presentation at the Institute of Medicine Conference on the Causes and Impacts of Neglected Tropical and Zoonotic Diseases, Washington, DC, September 22, 2010.

[94] Allison Garland and Lauren Herzer, "Water for the Urban Poor: Integrated Solutions," *SAIS Review*, vol. 29, no. 1 (Winter-Spring 2009), pp. 101-107.

[95] Japan, for example, addresses soil-transmitted helminths through the Hashimoto Initiative that operates in Thailand, Ghana, and Kenya.

[96] "Chair's Summary," G8 Summit, Hokkaido Toyako, Japan, July 9, 2008.

[97] Britain's Department of International Development, "£50 Million to Wipe Out Deadly Tropical Diseases ," press release, September 22, 2008.

[98] Netherlands Ministry of Foreign Affairs, *PDP Fund Against Poverty-Related Diseases*, Grants Order, May 21, 2010.

[99] Peter Hotez, "Neglected Tropical Disease Control in the "Post-American World"," *PLoS Neglected Tropical Diseases*, vol. 4, no. 8 (August 2010), e812.

[100] Katherine Bliss et al., *Key Players in Global Health: How Brazil, Russia, India, China, and South Africa Are Influencing the Game*, Center for Strategic International Studies, Washington, DC, November 2010.

[101] Peter Hotez, "Neglected Tropical Disease Control in the "Post-American World"," *PLoS Neglected Tropical Diseases*, vol. 4, no. 8 (August 2010), e812.

[102] The other four strategies are: MDA, intensified case-management, vector control, and the provision of safe water, sanitation and hygiene. See WHO, *First WHO Report on Neglected Tropical Diseases*, 2010, p. vii

[103] WHO webpage on NTDs, at http://www.who.int/neglected_diseasesneglected_diseases/faq/en/index.html.

[104] Webpage on the Global Network for Neglected Tropical Diseases at http://globalnetwork.org/.

[105] Webpage on the NTD Program at http://www.neglecteddiseases.gov/about/index.html.

[106] See the Global Alliance's webpage at http://www.filariasis.org/.

[107] The three onchocerciasis programs are eliminated in different regions, but all target blindness caused by onchocerciasis; see http://www.who.int/blindness/partnerships/onchocerciasis_home/en/index.html.

[108] For more information on the Schistosomiasis Control Initiative, see http://www3.imperial.ac.uk/schisto.

[109] For more information on the PPC, see http://www.who.int/wormcontrol/about_us/en/.

[110] For more information on GET 2020, see http://www.who.int/blindness/ causes/trachoma/en/index.html.

[111] For more information on the Trachoma Initiative, see http://www.trachoma

[112] WHO, *Chagas disease: control and elimination*, Report by the Secretariat, March 20, 2009, http://apps.who.int/gb/ebwha/pdf_files/A62/A62_17-en.pdf.

[113] WHO, *The Final Push Strategy to Eliminate Leprosy as a Public Health Problem*, Questions and Answers, 2003, http://www.who.int/lep/resources

[114] Jai Narain et al., "Elimination of neglected tropical diseases in the South-East Asia Region of the World Health Organization," *Bulletin of the World Health Organization*, vol. 88, no. 3 (2010), pp. 206-210, http://www.who.int/bulletin/volumes/88/3/09-072322/en/.

[115] See the Bill & Melinda Gates Foudnation webpage on NTDs at http://www.gatesfoundation.org/topics/Pages/ neglected-diseases.aspx.

[116] Bill & Melinda Gates Foundation, Neglected and Other Infectious Diseases, Strategy Overview, November 2009, http://www.gatesfoundation.org/global-health

[117] See the Carter Center webpage at http://www.cartercenter.org/index.html.

[118] http://www.childrenwithoutworms.org/.

[119] http://www.dndi.org/.

[120] See the Global Network webpage at http://www.globalnetwork.org/.

[121] See the International Vaccine Institute webpage at http://www.ivi.int/.

[122] See R. Dipika Sur et al., "A Cluster-Randomized Effectiveness Trial of Vi Typhoid Vaccine in India," *New England Journal of Medicine*, vol. 361, no. 4 (July 23, 2009), pp. 335-344, http://www.nejm.org/doi/pdf/10.1056/NEJMoa0807521.

[123] See the webpage of IDRI at http://www.idri.org/.

[124] See the Institute for One World Health webpage at http://www.oneworldhealth.org/about_us.

[125] Merck & Co., Inc., Corporate Social Responsibility 2008 Report, p. 19, http://www.merck.com/responsibility/ MRK2008CRReport.pdf.

[126] See the Sabin Institute webpage at http://www.sabin.org/.

[127] See the TDR webpage at http://apps.who.int/tdr/.

[128] TDR, *TDR Business Plan 2008-2013*, June 2007, p. 5, http://apps.who.int/tdr/documents/TDR-business-plan-2008.pdf. An *eliminated* disease no longer causes illness among a population, though the germ that causes the illness remains. In contrast, *eradication* ensures the causative agent is destroyed and the disease no longer causes illness.

[129] Ibid., *TDR Summary Report 2004*: *Covering years 2003-2004*, p. 9, http://apps.who.int/tdr/publications/about-tdr/summary-reports/summary-report-04/pdf/summary-report-04.pdf.

[130] Ibid., "TDR financial contributions 2008-2009," http://apps.who.int/tdr/about/pdf/contributions_table_2008_2009.pdf.

In: Neglected Tropical Diseases
Editor: Ronald J. Davidson
ISBN: 978-1-61324-387-9

Chapter 2

NEGLECTED TROPICAL DISEASES: IDENTIFYING RESEARCH GAPS AND OPPORTUNITIES*

National Institutes of Health
National Institute of Allergy and Infectious Diseases
Division of Microbiology and Infectious Diseases

Report of Workshop Held on September 27, 2007

Tropical diseases have been part of the NIH mission since its founding and are incorporated into the Public Health Service Act as part of the NIH mission. International collaborative efforts as well as public-private partnerships are generating new opportunities for making substantial progress in novel interventions for many infectious diseases of the tropics. Growing public interest in global health could add to this momentum. International efforts in malaria, tuberculosis and HIV are providing an infrastructure that overlaps geographically with endemic areas for many other infectious diseases, creating prospects for shared research capabilities and opportunities. The availability of new methodological approaches such as genomics,

---

* This is an edited, reformatted and augmented version of a National Institutes of Health's publication, dated September 27, 2007.

proteomics, synthetic chemistry, molecular and genetic epidemiology, as well as increases in information and communication technologies, may further enhance prospects for progress in research on many infectious diseases found in the tropics. Although many such diseases have been historically thought of as resulting from poverty, they have been more recently recognized as a significant cause of poverty that must be addressed in order to break the cycle of poverty.

Comparative Burden of Infectious Diseases in Disability Adjusted Life Years (DALYs)

	DALYs (millions)
Lower respiratory infections	91.4
HIV/AIDS	84.5
Diarrheal diseases	62.0
Neglected tropical diseases	56.6
Malaria	46.5
Tuberculosis	34.7
Measles	21.4

Source: WHO; Hotez, *et al.* N Engl J Med. 2007 Sep 6; 357(10):1018-27.

Neglected tropical diseases (NTDs) are a group of conditions that are among the most common infections in the world's most impoverished individuals. These diseases are caused by parasitic worms, protozoa, and bacteria, and primarily affect low income countries throughout sub-Saharan Africa, Asia, and Latin America. The majority of these diseases are transmitted by insect vectors, including mosquitoes, black flies, sand flies, and tsetse flies. Others are spread by contaminated water or soil infested with worms. While NTDs can be fatal, most often they result in chronic disabilities leading to disfigurements, impaired development, complications in pregnancy, and ultimately loss of worker productivity. In fact, NTDs rank closely with diarrheal diseases and malaria in the number of years lost to disability and premature death, or disability adjusted life-years (DALYs). Thus, NTDs perpetuate poverty by placing huge burdens on both the health and economic development of low-income countries. While treatments for some NTDs are available, many are not well tolerated by patients and have significant adverse side effects. The need for new interventions to prevent and treat these diseases becomes even more urgent in light of limited access to existing treatments, rapid reinfection following treatment, and drug resistance. (WHO; Global Network for Neglected Tropical Diseases; Hotez, *et al.* N Engl J Med. 2007 Sep 6; 357(10)1018-27)

Despite the burden of disease, research progress in NTDs lags behind many other infectious diseases. Research progress has been greatly hampered due to a number of obstacles, including:

- complex pathogen life cycles that are laborious and often expensive to maintain in the laboratory
- limited molecular tools for genetic manipulation and analysis on a genome-wide scale
- limited animal models of infection that mimic the human disease

At NIH, the National Institute of Allergy and Infectious Diseases (NIAID) supports basic and applied research to better understand, treat, and ultimately prevent infectious diseases, such as NTDs. In order to better understand current NTD research gaps and opportunities, the Division of Microbiology and Infectious Diseases (DMID) within the NIAID convened a workshop of leading experts in the various fields of NTD research.

Meeting participants were charged with addressing the following questions:

- What are the most important current research gaps in NTDs research and how can these best be addressed?
- What are the current barriers to research on NTDs and how might these be overcome?
- Which research areas are most promising in terms of identifying and advancing development of new strategies to combat NTDs?
- Are there overlapping areas of research and synergies that could have an impact on multiple NTDs?

To address these questions, invited experts first provided disease-focused presentations for each of the NTD pathogens listed in the table above. During these presentations, the experts provided a technical, non-prioritized description of research gaps and resource needs for each parasite. A summary of these presentations are presented in the *Pathogen Specific Areas* section in the appendix of this report.

Following these disease-focused presentations, the NTDs were separated into three pathogen focus areas for discussion: Protozoa, Helminth and

Bacteria. Meeting attendees were divided into discussion groups according to expertise and charged with identifying research priorities in immediate, intermediate and long-term time frames for these pathogen groups and the vectors that transmit them. These priorities as well as general background information on individual diseases are presented in the *Research Priorities within Pathogen Groups* section of this report.

As these diseases share many common obstacles that have hampered research progress, a number of cross- cutting areas became apparent through presentations and discussions at the meeting. See the *Cross Cutting Areas* section of this report for a summary.

The neglected tropical diseases (NTDs) discussed in this workshop:

- Protozoa
  Trypanosomiasis
  Leishmaniasis
- Helminth
  Schistosomiasis
  Filariasis
  Hookworm Soil-transmitted nematode infections
- Bacteria

Trachoma
Leprosy
Buruli ulcer

Research Priorities within Pathogen Groups

Protozoa (Trypanosoma and Leishmania)

Parasitic protozoa are single-celled organisms that cause a variety of debilitating and life-threatening diseases in humans. Species of parasitic protozoa from two genera, *Trypanosoma* and *Leishmania*, are responsible for diseases in the NTD group discussed at this meeting.

Protozoa in the genus *Trypanosoma* cause two types of diseases in humans: African sleeping sickness and Chagas' disease. *African trypanosomiasis* (sleeping sickness) is caused by *Trypanosoma brucei gambiense* and *Trypanosoma brucei rhodesiense* and is transmitted by the tsetse fly (*Glossina* spp.). An estimated 60 million people in 36 countries in sub-Saharan Africa are at risk for African trypanosomiasis, with an estimated 50,00070,000 people infected (http://www.who.int/mediacentre/ factsheets/ fs259/en/). Sleeping sickness is invariably fatal if left untreated, and available treatments produce severe side effects in some patients. Major epidemics are a constant threat to the economic development of Central and East Africa.

American trypanosomiasis (Chagas' disease) is caused by *Trypanosoma cruzi* and is transmitted by insects commonly known as "kissing bugs" of the subfamily *Triatominae* (Family *Reduviidae*). The acute phase of the disease following infection may last for a few weeks or months and often goes undetected. Untreated cases, however, may develop into chronic infections leading to damage to the nervous system, digestive system, and heart. An estimated 100 million people are at risk in 21 countries in Central and South America with 16-18 million people infected. There are 1 million new cases of chronic disease and more than 45,000 deaths annually. (http://www.who.int/ tdr/diseases

Leishmaniasis is caused by protozoa in the genus *Leishmania* (20 species are pathogenic for humans) and is transmitted by the phlebotomine sandfly. An estimated 350 million people are at risk in 88 countries with 12 million people infected. There are three basic forms of the disease: cutaneous, mucocutaneous, and visceral. Cutaneous leishmaniasis, the most common form of the disease, results in non-healing, scaling lesions of the skin that often ulcerate and become infected secondarily with bacteria. Mucocutaneous leishmaniasis affects mucous membranes and produces destructive and often disfiguring lesions of the face. In visceral leishmaniasis (also known as kala-azar), the most severe form of the disease, the parasite infects internal organs such as the liver, spleen and bone marrow, resulting in death if left untreated. More than 90 percent of the world's cases of visceral leishmaniasis are in India, Bangladesh, Nepal, Sudan, and Brazil. In addition, the incidence of HIV/*Leishmania* co-infections is increasing, especially in southern Europe. (http://www.who.int/leishmaniasis/burden/en/)

Protozoa Research Priorities
[Leishmania spp., Trypanosoma cruzi, Trypanosoma brucei]

Immediate Priorities	Intermediate Priorities	Long Term Priorities
• Basic Science • Database Development	• Molecular Tools • Diagnostics and Biomarkers	• Drug Development • Field Site

Immediate Priorities

For specific information on basic science research gaps, please see the Pathogen-Specific Areas section. Identifying new drug targets and developing animal models for drug evaluation (especially for *T. cruzi* and *Leishmania* parasites) are important due to the relatedness of these organisms, and a comprehensive comparison of Trypanosomatid genomes could provide important insights. For example, such comparative efforts could identify genes important for pathogenicity that are common to all three parasites, and functional studies could then be pursued in *T. brucei*, the only parasite for which genetic manipulation is currently feasible. Host immune responses to parasites may contribute either to protection or to pathology, and the molecular correlates of these responses remains unknown. Similarly, interventions that modulate the host's immune response so as to enhance protection and mitigate pathology may be beneficial. *Leishmania* and *T. cruzi* are intracellular parasites, meaning they spend a significant portion of their life cycles residing inside human cells. A greater understanding of this intracellular phase may provide important insights relevant to evasion of host immune responses and parasite metabolism that in turn could lead to the identification and development of novel antiparasitic interventions.

Insect vectors are responsible for transmission of these protozoan parasites. As such, basic science research on the biology of insect vectors is an important priority, particularly research aimed at identifying vector molecules essential for parasite growth and development in the insect. Additionally, improved methods of vector population management, such as paratransgenesis, are important for disease control. (Paratransgenesis is a technique that modifies symbiotic microbes living within the vector to produce molecules that prevent disease transmission.)

Databases, such as GeneDB, are needed in order to integrate and organize available information (e.g. genomic data) for use by the community. Such databases may increase understanding of parasite gene function leading to the identification of unique targets for drug and diagnostic development. Because the value of such databases is dependent on the extent to which the scientific community utilizes them, community involvement in database development and maintenance will be important.

Intermediate Priorities

Improved molecular tools are important for investigating the function of predicted genes. Such tools may include:

- cloned sets of gene sequences ("open reading frames") that code for proteins, as well as the means ("shuttle vectors") to express proteins based on such sequences in various systems; and
- high-throughput studies of gene function using RNA-interference (RNAi) to systematically shut down each parasite gene in order to identify the necessary components of a particular cellular process.

Information obtained from the use of the molecular tools described above may lead to the identification of new *biomarkers,* molecular indicators of the presence of infection or the extent of disease. Such markers can form the basis for development of new *diagnostics* to determine the same. Furthermore, biomarkers can be used to monitor insect vector populations in the field for species identification, pathogen presence, and insecticide resistance.

Long Term Priorities

Drug development leading to new treatment options is important as currently available drugs are expensive, limited in number, and often toxic. In addition, parasite resistance to existing drugs in increasingly common. Field sites are essential for research efforts on a number of NTDs. However, more than one disease may be present at the same location. Thus, in the future *field site capacity in endemic areas* should include expertise in multiple disease areas for treatment, vaccination and vector management. Where co-morbidity exists, coordination to understand the effects of managing multiple diseases is possible. Since these pathogens are transmitted via insect vectors, increased *vector research* is also important, particularly with respect to vector competence and vector/pathogen interactions. To optimize the impact of these research activities, it will be important to establish a dialog with disease control programs so that research findings and new interventions can be incorporated into control efforts in a timely fashion.

Helminth Infections (Schistosomiasis, Filariasis, Hookworm, and Related Infections)

Parasitic worms are among the most common causes of chronic human infections worldwide – particularly schistosomiasis, filariasis, onchocerciasis and intestinal roundworm infections. *Schistosomiasis* is caused by trematode flatworms of the genus *Schistosoma.* An estimated 600 million people are at risk in 74 countries with 200 million infected. While mortality remains relatively low, tens of millions have debilitating chronic morbidity. (http://www.who.int/schistosomiasis/en/)

Lymphatic filariasis (elephantiasis) is caused by the parasitic filarial worms *Wuchereria bancrofti* and *Brugia malayi.* An estimated 1.2 billion people are at risk in 83 countries throughout the tropics and sub-tropics of Asia, Africa, the Western Pacific, and parts of the Caribbean and South America. An estimated 120 million people are infected worldwide with at least 40 million people severely affected with hydrocoele, lymphedema or sub-clinical lymphatic damage. (http://www.who.int/mediacentre/factsheets/fs102/en/index.html)

Onchocerciasis (river blindness) is caused by the filarial worm *Onchocerca volvulus* and is transmitted through the bites of infected black flies of the *Simulium* species. The disease is prevalent in 30 countries of Africa, 13 countries in the Americas (including Mexico, Guatemala, Ecuador, Colombia, Venezuela, and Brazil) and in Yemen. Worldwide, there are around 18 million people infected and 270,000 people who have become blind as a consequence of long-term infection. (http://www.cdc.gov/ncidod/dpd/parasites/onchocerciasis/factsht onchocerciasis.htm)

Intestinal helminth (roundworm) infections are among the most common human infections, especially in tropical and sub-tropical countries, and are the leading cause of disease burden in children aged 5 to 14 years. Worldwide, 1.5 billion people are infected with *Ascaris* (http://www.cdc.gov/ncidod/dpd/parasites/ascaris/factsht ascaris.htm), 800 million with *Trichuris* (http://www.dpd.cdc.gov/DPDx/HTML/Trichuriasis.htm) and 1.3 billion with hookworms (http://www.cdc.gov/ncidod/dpd/parasites/hookwormhookworm.htm). Moderate infections are associated with poor physical and mental development, while more intense infections can result in severe anemia (hookworms), intestinal obstruction (ascariasis), and chronic colitis (trichuriasis).

Helminth Research Priorities [Schistosoma spp., Filarial worms, Hookworms, Soil-Transmitted Nematodes]

Immediate Priorities	Intermediate Priorities	Long Term Priorities
• Basic Science • Diagnostics and Biomarkers • Drug Development • Clinical Studies • Reagents and Materials Resources • Database Development	• Diagnostics and Biomarkers • Reagents and Materials Resources • Drug Development • Clinical Studies • Database Development	• Diagnostics • Drug Development • Vaccine Development

Immediate Priorities

For specific information on *basic scien***ce** research gaps, please see the *Pathogen-Specific Areas* section.

Improved *diagnostics* are important for helminth infections because they are essential for assessing epidemiologic aspects of these diseases and enhancing the effectiveness of ongoing global control or elimination programs. Further, vaccine and drug development efforts must detect and quantify active infection at an early stage. To address this need, attention should be directed at the following:

- new target diagnostic molecules (*biomarkers*) that identify the infecting pathogen
- diagnostic markers that will aid in monitoring vector populations and their rates of infection
- increasing the sensitivity of existing assays, particularly through the use of new test platforms

Drugs are currently being used in global health programs targeting more than half a billion people each year, yet each of these programs relies on only one or two effective drugs. With the ever present threat of parasitic worms developing resistance to these drugs and with therapeutic profiles (i.e., the combination of efficacy and toxicity) of available drugs being less than ideal, potential new drugs need to be identified. Genomic and proteomic tools offer new opportunities to identify new drug targets and to define mechanisms of action for currently used drugs. Such knowledge could provide a firm scientific rationale for all research efforts to detect resistance and to develop new drugs. Use of both *in vivo* models and high-throughput screens are essential for early-stage studies to screen for new drugs, to establish proof-of-principle, and eventually to advance new leads into pre-clinical drug-development studies.

Clinical Studies provide opportunities to define currently unanticipated effects of co-infections on expected therapeutic outcomes or vaccine responses and to define strategies to prevent potential adverse effects. Specifically, there is a dearth of information on the following:

- co-infections, in which one infection has the potential to affect the pathogenesis and clinical outcome of another co-morbid disease
- individualized responses to WHO's Expanded Program on Immunization (EPI) or other vaccines as a result of helminth co-infections
- multi-drug treatment interventions and their effects on the therapeutic outcomes of coincident infections

Because of the complexity of life cycles, the limited range of animal models, and the restricted opportunities for researchers (particularly those in the U.S. or Europe) to work with patients with helminth NTDs, *reagents and materials resources* including repositories of the relevant parasite, vector and human specimens are important to maintain scientific progress. Indeed, as noted by meeting participants, the availability over the past four decades of NIAID-supported resource repositories has proven essential for much of the successful research in both filariasis and schistosomiasis.

Databases that effectively integrate and organize available information (e.g. genomic data, reagents and materials resources) for use by the community could greatly advance research efforts on helminth parasites.

Intermediate Priorities

Improved *diagnostics,* such as point-of-care (POC) assays, that require only small amounts of sample material and are suitable for use in field sites would be especially valuable for field research and use in large-scale control programs. New proteomic/genomic approaches can be used to identify diagnostic targets for use in POC assays that would both detect and quantify active infection. Once validated, these new assays could also be used for routine screening of asymptomatic individuals for the presence of these parasites. *Biomarkers,* including the small metabolic products of infecting parasites and infected hosts, can now be studied through techniques such as high-throughput mass spectroscopy and new microarray assays. Studies of host and pathogen biomarkers have the potential to identify states of disease progression, protection afforded by experimental vaccines, and even pre-symptomatic infection.

Increased development of *reagents and materials resources* is important for the storage and distribution of well-characterized field specimens from individuals with different disease stages. Such a resource would greatly facilitate research on infections caused by helminths.

Continued development of lead compounds affecting potential targets identified in earlier studies is a priority. Chemistry resources will be essential for modifying lead candidates through computational and synthetic approaches. For promising candidates, capacity for formulation, production scale-up, and safety and toxicity testing will be useful.

Clinical studies offer opportunities to investigate unique and important aspects of these diseases, some of which may have broader implications, such as:

- the interrelation of host responses to helminth infection and environmental allergens as both result in elevated immunoglobulin E (IgE) antibodies, suggesting that immune responses in these conditions share common elements
- the effect of molecules produced or induced by these parasites during the course of infection
    - vasoactive molecules – those capable of dilating or constricting blood vessels
    - anticoagulant molecules – those capable of preventing blood clotting

The maintenance of *databases* should be on-going and, optimally, expanded to allow increasing research opportunities and needs to be addressed in a timely manner.

Long Term Priorities

Development of rapid, sensitive, quantitative, and inexpensive point-of-care diagnostics (as described above) is important to support clinical studies of new interventions. Long-term support of *drug* development will be critical for advancing drug candidates further into Phase I clinical trials, with the potential of Phase II trials and beyond. In view of the potential for pathogens to develop resistance to widely deployed drugs, it is important to develop and maintain a robust pipeline of new antihelminthic therapeutics. Current mathematical modeling of transmission and disease prevention supports the importance of a schistosomiasis *vaccine* that could ultimately be used in conjunction with drug therapy. In the zoonotic setting of disease caused by *Schistosoma japonicum*, a vaccine for animal use might also be important. A similar rationale exists for the filarial diseases (lymphatic filariaris [LF] or *Onchocerca volvulus* [OV]).

Bacteria (Trachoma and Mycobacterial Infections)

Buruli ulcer is caused by infection with *Mycobacterium ulcerans* and can result in extensive skin ulcerations, which are typically found on an infected individual's arms or legs. If not treated early, the ulcerations can cause extensive skin and soft tissue destruction that often leads to the restriction of joint movement, and in time, the patient may require limb amputation. There is evidence that *M. ulcerans* is not transmitted person to person but is an environmental mycobacterium that is likely transmitted to humans from aquatic environments, small aquatic animals and biofilms. Humans appear to have increased risk of infection in areas with stagnant or slow moving water, but the mode of transmission is still under investigation. While disease has been reported in 30 countries, the extent of disease within these countries is not known. (http://www.who.int/buruli/en/)

Leprosy (Hansen's Disease) is a chronic infectious disease that affects skin, nervous tissue, respiratory tract, and eyes and is caused by infection with *Mycobacterium leprae*. While treatment is available in early stages of the disease, there is no treatment once nerves are damaged. *M. leprae* is capable of causing a wide range of clinical manifestations including peripheral neurological damage (nerve damage in the arms and legs), which causes *sensory loss* in the skin as well as muscle *weakness*. People with long-term infection may lose the use of their hands or feet due to repeated traumatic injury resulting from lack of sensation. The stigma long associated with leprosy still exists in many parts of the world and the psychological and social stigma may be more difficult to deal with than the actual physical illness that it causes. Recent trends in Hansen's Disease epidemiology suggest a decline in the actual number of cases. The number of new cases detected annually has raised questions about the source of infection, transmission, and incubation period of *M. leprae*. (http://www.who.int/lep/en/)

Trachoma is an infection of the eye caused by the bacterium *Chlamydia trachomatis* and is the leading cause of preventable blindness in the world. Trachoma presents as a chronic inflammation of the conjunctiva that in turn can cause scarring of the conjunctiva and cornea, leading to blindness. Chronic, repeat infections occur most often in children under 10 years of age. Approximately 11 million cases of infection and 8 million cases of blindness occur annually worldwide. Trachoma is endemic in the poorest regions of Africa, Asia and the Middle East, and in some parts of South America and Australia. (http://www.who.int/blindness/causes/priority/en/index2.html)

Bacterial NTD Research Priorities
[*Mycobacterium leprae, Mycobacterium ulcerans, Chlamydia trachomatis*]

Immediate Priorities	Intermediate and Long Term Priorities
• Basic Science • Drug Development • Field Site Capacity in Endemic Areas • Reagents and Materials Resources	• Diagnostics • Vaccine Development

Immediate Priorities

For specific information on basic science research gaps, please see the Pathogen-Specific Areas section.

The development of drugs effective against trachoma and mycobacterial infections is important. Possible strategies may include:

- a safe, non-injectable drug therapeutic regimen for *M. ulcerans* using existing antibiotics approved for other infections
- assessment of antibiotic resistance in *M. leprae* by using clinical isolates from multiple regions of the world where leprosy is prevalent
- establishing community-wide antibiotic regimens for trachoma treatment and elimination programs and applying results to develop mathematical models for other community-wide programs

As field sites are critical for NTD research, building and enhancing *field site capacity in endemic areas* represent important priorities for these bacterial diseases. Improving integration of international research efforts with developing country laboratories would also be helpful. As an example, this could involve developing and maintaining resources to provide critical materials to developing country laboratories (*e.g.,* the armadillo model for growing *M. leprae*). These laboratories could reciprocate by providing certified clinical reagents and other specimens for use in international research efforts.

Increased development of *reagents and materials resources* is also important, including repositories of the relevant parasite and human specimens, such as those provided by the Leprosy Research Support program (see *NIAID Resources* section).

Intermediate and Long Term Priorities

Biomarkers are molecular indicators of the presence of infection. Such markers can form the basis for *diagnostics* development to determine the presence of infection or the extent of disease progression. Development of such *diagnostics* is important, including point-of-care (POC) assays that are rapid and employ a common platform for use with multiple chemical components and organisms.

Vaccine Development is also a possibility for these bacterial infections. One strategy would be to identify epitopes, or parts of molecules unique to these bacteria that are recognized by the human immune system, that may be useful for vaccine development. The large scale study of bacterial proteins (proteomics), particularly their structures, may aid in identifying these unique epitopes. Further, such epitopes may be identified from biomarkers used in development of diagnostics.

Cross-Cutting Areas

Diagnostics and Biomarkers

Improved diagnostics and biomarkers were identified as important research priorities for a number of NTDs. Diagnostics are needed to identify infected patients for treatment, to conduct surveillance of treatment effectiveness, and for assessing outcomes in drug and vaccine efficacy trials. Diagnostics and biomarkers should be able to identify active infection as well as stage or form of disease. Ideally, assays for related or multiple NTDs might be performed on the same platform so as to simplify infrastructure needs as well as to allow for testing for multiple agents in areas where co-infections commonly occur. Nanotechnology and other new technologies may lead to new platforms at the micro-level and thus allow for maximum usage of limited specimen materials. High-throughput screens may provide an efficient method to identify new diagnostic targets in the pathogens and markers for monitoring vector populations in the field.

Database and Computational Resources

Databases of genomic-related information that are curated and regularly updated as well as tools/software that can be used to access and query them were identified as important research priorities for a number of NTDs. In order to avoid duplication of efforts, databases should contain information on approaches (*e.g.*, drug targets) that have proven unsuccessful as well as those that have succeeded. Databases might also include a list of specimens (parasites, vectors, DNA, etc.) available in repositories that have been well characterized and can be used for a variety of purposes. These resources are anticipated to facilitate progress in developing diagnostics, biomarkers, drugs, and vaccines by identifying host or infectious agent proteins that are upregulated in specific disease states.

Reagent/Materials Resources

Resource centers that can readily distribute and collect materials nationally and internationally are important for research on all NTDs, and continued support for existing resource centers for filariasis, schistosomiasis, and leprosy was identified as a priority by meeting participants. It is also important to maintain well-characterized field specimens (including the range of pathogenic forms of individual diseases) that are made available through resource repositories and are included as part of a database for field studies. Research materials such as whole infectious organisms or organism components (especially for difficult to maintain/prepare organisms) are useful, as are reagents such as monoclonal antibodies, recombinant clones, and microarrays. In addition to parasite-specific microarrays, microarrays that include genes from multiple parasites as well as the human host could prove beneficial for research efforts.

Field Resources

Several groups noted that multi-functional sites that serve as shared field resources could greatly benefit the field. Such sites could be used to gather clinically validated specimens for use in diagnostic and biomarker development. They could be used to study co-morbidity issues and to assess preventive or therapeutic interventions. Field sites are also essential for developing vector management strategies, and personnel at such sites can serve as resources for a variety of intervention studies. Efforts to incorporate research capacity into program intervention sites should be considered as a cost-effective way to both conduct research and assess the effectiveness of public health/program interventions. As appropriate, efforts to interface with large-scale international programs aimed at malaria, TB, and HIV research, should also be considered. For example, informed consent strategies could be developed that anticipate the use of specimens over the long term and as new research issues arise or technologies become available.

Drug Development

For all NTD organisms, development of new or better drugs is a research priority as is an approach based on rational drug design, in which structural information about targets is used as the basis for creating new drugs. For many NTDs, limited drug regimens are available and may be toxic. Without a larger, more diverse arsenal of drug therapies, there is an increased risk for organisms to develop resistance against the few existing drugs.

Genomic information and high-throughput screening are likely to facilitate identification of new drug targets. Studies are ongoing to screen drugs approved for alternative indications for activity against NTDs. This work should continue and, if resources permit, be expanded. Parasitic infections have complex effects on human physiology, thus as an added benefit, parasite products may serve as the basis for drug development for non-parasitic diseases, *e.g.*, as immune modulators, vasculature modulators, or anticoagulants. Further, improved animal models are important for many NTDs in order to facilitate preclinical drug development efforts.

Vaccine Development

Prophylactic vaccines may not be viable for NTDs of low incidence or prevalence; however, with the immunopathology associated with many NTDs, these diseases might be appropriate targets for therapeutic vaccines. Additionally, for diseases that are also present in an animal reservoir, there is potential to reduce disease incidence in humans indirectly by vaccinating these animals. Animal hosts could also serve as proof-ofprinciple for developing human vaccines. When designing such vaccines, scientists should consider characteristics of target populations and possible treatment modalities (preventive versus therapeutic).

Basic Research Issues

"Molecular toolboxes" for NTDs were identified as an important research priority by many of the groups. While this may vary by infectious agent, the basic concept involves common methodologies for genetic manipulations (*e.g.*, RNAi, recombinant vectors for gene knockouts). For all the NTDs, it is important to better understand the molecular basis of pathogenesis. For example, determinants of the different clinical forms of Chagas' disease are not known, and the roles of toxins in bacterial NTDs are not fully understood. Knowledge in these areas would enhance the ability to develop treatment strategies such as drugs and therapeutic vaccines as well as to define diagnostics and biomarkers. As many NTDs are transmitted by invertebrate vectors, a greater understanding of the interaction between vector and parasite is also important. Such research may be useful to identify potential targets for parasite growth and survival within the vector and transmission to the human host.

Clinical Research Issues

Defining clinical correlates for protective immune responses and surrogate markers for disease pathogenesis or resolution were identified as research priorities. Furthermore, defining the "infectome", *i.e.*, the array of genes preferentially expressed during the disease state, for individual stages of disease as well as for the infectious agent and its vector would be useful. The infectome includes correlates of microbial pathogenesis, and changes in the expression of genes in the infectome may provide insights into both host and microbial responses to therapy. This knowledge is important to develop and assess preventive and therapeutic strategies. It may also help to elucidate the role of host genetic factors in susceptibility, resistance, and response to infection, as well as the effects of vector saliva on the pathogenesis of the parasite in the human host. Further, it is important to determine the effects of co-infections and/or multiple treatments on the pathogenesis of an immune response to NTDs. Likewise, the effect of multiple infections on responses to candidate NTD drugs and vaccines should be determined. Clinical trials require research infrastructure and field sites, and there is the potential to coordinate NTD trials with facilities that are participating in studies of malaria, tuberculosis, HIV or other infectious diseases.

Mathematical Models

As interventional studies are designed, consideration should be given to collecting data and information that could be used to validate mathematical models of disease intervention strategies. It would be beneficial if extant empiric data could be made available to mathematicians to develop and test models.

Investigator Base

A "critical mass" of investigators is essential for progress in any research endeavor. Strategies to attract and retain new investigators for NTD research need to be explored, especially given the high degrees of complexity of carrying out research in these diseases that may deter investigators from entering or staying in the field.

Funding Opportunities

Investigators should be made aware of the variety of mechanisms and funding sources that may support their research goals. This is especially true for international collaborative efforts. In order to assure the relevance and appropriateness of proposed research, it would be beneficial if study sections reviewing applications on high priority translational research topics (e.g., diagnostics) included specialized expertise and familiarity with NTDs.

Collaborative Opportunities

When possible, research efforts could be coordinated to enhance targeted, cost-effective goals. Better communication between basic researchers and program/intervention investigators may be beneficial in accomplishing this. Control programs and research programs in individual NTDs could benefit from better linkages, and attempts to highlight such benefits and encourage such interactions should be made. Creative, ethical approaches to human subject issues need to be sought to facilitate harmonization between intervention programs and research. Solving complex problems, such as drug development and vector management strategies will require interdisciplinary research approaches, and where possible these should be facilitated.

NIAID Resources

Research Resources Relevant to NTDs

Activity	Resource/URL	Contact
Maintenance and supply of schistosome- infected snails and mammals through which investigators can obtain schistosome life stages. Three major schistosome species affecting humans (*S. mansoni*, *S. haematobium*, and *S. japonicum*) obtained either in their specific snail host, or in infected mammals.	NIAID Schistosomiasis Resource Center http://www.schisto-resource.org/	D. McGowan dmcgowan@niaid.nih.gov
The repository offers three filarial parasite species (*B. malayi, B. pahangi and D. immitis*). These parasites are maintained in the laboratory by alternate passage through mammalian definitive hosts and arthropod vectors. The Filariasis Repository Service includes molecular resources.	NIAID/NIH Filariasis Research Reagent Repository Center http://www.filariasiscenter.org/ Molecular Resources http://www.filariasiscenter.org/mole-center/index.htm	D. McGowan dmcgowan@niaid.nih.gov
Source of appreciable quantities of *M. leprae* and its various products.	Leprosy Research Support: http://www.cvmbs.colostate.edu/mip/leprosy/globalleprosy3.html	C. Sizemore csizemore@niaid.nih.gov

A complete listing of NIAID's research resources may be found at http://www.niaid.nih.gov/research/resources/.

Workshop Participants

Norma Andrews
Yale University School of Medicine
New Haven, Connecticut

Patrick Brennan Colorado State University
Fort Collins,
Colorado

Oscar Campetella
Universidad Nacional de General San Martin
Buenos Aires, Argentina

Dan Colley
University of Georgia Research Foundation,
Center for Tropical and Emerging Global Diseases
Athens, Georgia

Michael Cappello (in absentia)
Yale University
New Haven, Connecticut

John E. Donelson
University of Iowa
Iowa City, Iowa

Najib M. El-Sayed
University of Maryland
College Park, Maryland

Phil LoVerde
Southwest Foundation for Biomedical Research
San Antonio, Texas

James H. McKerrow
University of California, San Francisco
San Francisco, California

David M. Mosser
University of Maryland
College Park, Maryland

Eric A. Ottesen
Emory University
Atlanta, Georgia

Steven G. Reed
Infectious Disease Research Institute
Seattle, Washington

Julius Schachter
University of California,
San Francisco San Francisco, California

Pamela Small
University of Tennessee
Knoxville, Tennessee

Ken Stuart
Seattle Biomedical Research Institute
Seattle, Washington

Shyam Sundar
Banaras Hindu University
Institute of Medical Sciences
Varanasi, India

Rick L. Tarleton
University of Georgia
Athens, Georgia

Richard Truman
U.S. Public Health Service
National Hansen's Disease Program
at Louisiana State University
Baton Rouge, Louisiana

Sergio Verjovski-Almeida
Universidade de Sao Paulo
Sao Paulo, Brazil

Sheila K. West
Johns Hopkins University
Baltimore, Maryland

Steve Williams
Smith College
Northampton, Massachusetts

APPENDIX: PROCEEDINGS FROM WORKING GROUPS ON SPECIFIC PATHOGENS

Meeting participants were divided into three discussion groups based on expertise to prioritize research goals for the NTDs discussed. The immediate, intermediate, and long-term goals for each pathogen group (protozoa, helminth, and bacteria) are described in the main body of this report. This appendix contains a more technical, non-prioritized listing of research gaps and resource needs for each pathogen.

Protozoa

Trypanosoma Brucei

Basic Science Research Gaps

The genome for *Trypanosoma brucei* has been sequenced and is available electronically (http://www.tigr.org/tdb/e2k1/tba1/intro.shtml). Despite the availability of the genome, a function has not been assigned to the majority of predicted genes, and in cases where the function is known, the genes have been found to be highly divergent or unique. Thus, many challenges remain that would benefit from expanded efforts.

Diagnostics and Biomarkers

With the genetic relationship among Trypanosomatid organisms, there is an opportunity for using common technical approaches and exploiting the knowledge from bioinformatics and genomics to develop biomarkers that can be used to elucidate pathogenesis, to form the basis for point-of-care diagnostics, and to confirm infection for treatment with currently available drugs and/or enrollment of participants in drug trials. These biomarkers encompass pathogen and host, including host immune responses. In conjunction with this effort, validated clinical and field samples (and possibly some experimental samples) for developing and testing diagnostics and biomarkers is important. Access to analytical resources, such as mass spectrometry, protein arrays and immunoassays, is another component required for this work. Developing appropriate platforms is necessary; information on the kinds of platforms available should be provided to the research community. A repository for materials essential for development of diagnostics and biomarkers would be beneficial, especially for materials that are already available and developed in specific research labs, such as cloned gene sequences, monoclonal antibodies, and recombinant vectors. Markers for monitoring vector populations in the field are also crucial, including vector species identification, pathogen presence and insecticide resistance.

Target Identification and Candidate Therapeutics

Drug development requires multiple disciplines and the exploration of multiple drug targets. The unique metabolism of the trypanosomes, the fact that 25 percent of the genome encodes protein enzymes, and the close genetic relationship of the Trypanosomatid protozoa may provide unique opportunities for therapeutics in terms of targets and classes of compounds. As in the genome projects for these organisms, community coordination will be beneficial.

Vaccines

Vaccines are not a priority for *T. brucei*, as antigenic variation makes prophylactic vaccines unlikely. However, there is a remote possibility for the development of therapeutic vaccines, which may alleviate the suffering of infected individuals. Further, transmission blocking vaccines may also be considered including strategies for targeting the insect vector as well as animal reservoirs.

Disease Control

The Trypanosomatid diseases offer an opportunity to study the impact of multiple control measures in disease eradication/reduction including the coordinated use of drugs, insecticides, transmission blocking vaccines, etc. These measures may include management strategies that affect tsetse fly populations and contact with the human host. Knowledge gained from interventions in these diseases may also provide insights useful for other NTDs.

Trypanosoma Cruzi

Basic Science Research Gaps

There are numerous significant gaps in our knowledge of Chagas' disease. Whether clinical forms are associated with parasite and/or host genetic variation is unknown as are the fundamental molecular and cellular events that lead to organ enlargement and malfunction during the clinical course of infection. Also, little is known about the role of innate immunity in preventing establishment of infection, the mechanisms controlling the host's initial response to infection, the effect of treatment on the host's immunological memory and resistance to re-infection, the effect of length of infection on immune control, and the parasite mechanisms of immune evasion.

Target Identification and Candidate Therapeutics

The development of less toxic drugs and of drugs effective for treating patients during the chronic stage of *T. cruzi* infection is essential. Drug candidates currently in early stages of testing and development include protease inhibitors and anti-fungal triazoles. Development of new drugs could be enhanced by identifying biochemical pathways unique to the parasite, validating potential drug targets, developing screening assays, and testing libraries of compounds.

The limited arsenal of available drugs could be used more effectively by early disease detection leading to a shortened course of treatment. Such a strategy may decrease the rate of drug resistance. Placebo-controlled trials are key in demonstrating efficacy of chronic disease treatment.

Diagnostics and Biomarkers

It is important to determine whether additional specific tests can be developed for diagnosing infections. This is particularly important due to concerns about potential for contamination of the blood supply. Accurate diagnostics could address this problem. Furthermore, surrogate biomarkers for infection are critical for future assessments of vaccine effectiveness in preventing long-term sequelae, determining disease outcomes, and predicting therapeutic outcomes in drug treatment trials.

Host Response, Immunology, and Vaccines

A vaccine for humans may decrease the number of circulating organisms and therefore decrease transmission; however, this approach will not address animal reservoirs harboring parasites with human infective potential. Domestic animals living in close proximity to humans serve as parasite reservoirs, thus a vaccine developed for domestic animals would likely reduce transmission to humans indirectly. An acute phase vaccine for Chagas' disease may also be useful for preventing or controlling infection in children.

Resources

With respect to the genomics of American Trypanosomiasis, it is important to sequence, assemble and annotate additional non-hybrid isolates, to expand Expressed Sequence Tag (EST) databanks, to establish curated community-supported databases, and to identify biochemical pathways that are viable drug targets (*e.g.,* transsialidases, phosphokinases, genes involved in DNA replication/repair).

Vector Biology

A greater understanding of the molecular interactions that occur between *T.cruzi* parasites and the triatome gut, *e.g.,* the signals for differentiation of epimastigotes into infective trypomastigotes, is a priority. Studies on vector ecology and population structure are also necessary as is a better understanding of vector behavior. For example, it has been demonstrated that triatomines in the peridomestic environment come into contact with infected animals and humans and become involved in the human food chain. The significance of this behavior and its implications was demonstrated by the recent episodes of human *T. cruzi* infections following açai juice consumption in Brazil.

Leishmania species

Basic Science Research Gaps

Better use of the existing Leishmania genome sequences could accelerate progress in understanding basic processes of these parasites. A more complete understanding of the mechanism(s) of intracellular survival, including amastigote biology and the host's immunological response, will be crucial to future progress. . Furthermore, the molecular basis for chronicity of infections is not known and could be potentially aided by the development of animal models. Studies employing gene deletions in *Leishmania* spp. and RNAi in *L. braziliensis* could facilitate the functional characterization of genes of interest.

Host Response, Immunology, and Vaccines

Better understanding of the immunology of *Leishmania* infections, the genetics of human susceptibility and resistance, and the basis for the different disease forms (cutaneous, muco-cutaneous, and visceral) is key in facilitating *Leishmania* vaccine development. Additionally, the affect of sand fly saliva on the pathogenicity of different *Leishmania* species is important to understand.

Since dogs are also susceptible to *Leishmania* infections and serve as reservoirs, a vaccine for dogs may limit transmission as well as inform development of vaccines for human use. For example, Brazilian investigators are pursuing the concept of combining a *Leishmania* vaccine with a rabies vaccine for dogs as a way of controlling both diseases.

Leishmania vaccines have been tested internationally, including a heat-killed vaccine in Iran and therapeutic vaccines in Brazil and Sudan. If information can be made available about the specific results from such efforts in a timely manner, they may provide insights and potentially accelerate the further development of human vaccines. Efforts are also underway to develop a vaccine based on sand fly saliva proteins.

Vector Biology

As leishmaniasis is transmitted to humans via an insect vector, an increased knowledge of sand fly biology, ecology and behavior is an important priority. In addition, it is important to further define the molecular interactions between vector and parasite. Such research may lead to the development of new vector management strategies, insecticides and transmission blocking vaccines.

Target Identification and Candidate Therapeutics

Drug resistance and drug development are areas that would benefit from further investigation. Recent studies on Interleukin-10 and the pathogenesis of human visceral leishmaniasis suggest that future drugs and vaccines need both to target the parasite and manipulate the immune response.

Resources

Investigational resources are vital to progress and may include controllable and inducible expression systems that do not break down over time, large-scale knock-out systems that are readily usable for hundreds to thousands of genes, and other genetic tools such as the Cre-lox DNA recombination system and RNAi. Databases, similar to those available for yeast and *C. elegans*, which catalog available information (*e.g.* genomic data), are key to *Leishmania* research.

Helminth

Schistosoma species

Basic Science Research Gaps

It is important to better understand the immunology and pathology of schistosome infection (in human and in model systems), the effects of schistosome infection on the immune response system, the role of host genetic polymorphisms in resistance to disease and in morbidity, and the effect of drug treatment on the immune responses to disease.

Genomic and post-genomic technologies (including proteomics and glycomics) could be applied to schistosome life-cycle forms, to vector snail species as well as to organisms *in situ* and *ex vivo*. The goals would encompass the sequencing, annotation, and database development for both parasite and vector genomes, which would expedite comparisons of snail and parasite species and strains. It is anticipated that additional *Schistosoma* genomes will be available shortly, and *Biomphalaria glabrata* snail genome sequencing efforts are ongoing.

A better understanding of the basic biology of schistosome life-cycle stages may facilitate their use as a model parasite system. Increased research on schistosome fecundity and egg excretion, schistosome germ cells, host–parasite interactions, and the infected host's neurobiology and neuromuscular physiology will also provide useful information.

Developing a "molecular tool box" for schistosomes, including knockouts and transgenic lines, to allow and enhance studies of genes, molecules and organism functions through the life cycle stages is a priority. Biochemical and molecular studies, incorporating genomics, glycomics, and proteomics, can help elucidate schistosome membrane biology and metabolism during different life stages. Furthermore, it is important to better characterize functional roles and possible medical uses of molecules produced/released by shistosomes.

Diagnostics

It is important to optimize and combine existing diagnostic tools more effectively, including immunological assays that detect infection or assess disease status and ultrasound detection to evaluate pathology. Assays that measure worm burdens in active infection are also important as are diagnostic tools for detection of morbidity or pre-morbidity.

Transmission

Increased knowledge of the ecological and biological aspects of the snail vector would likely lead to greater understanding of the snail responses to schistosome infection, how these responses relate to differences in parasite strains and whether there are comparative differences in field *versus* laboratory parasite isolates. The influence of societal components on disease transmission is also an important area that may benefit from increased research. More information on transmission dynamics including mathematical models and the role of humans and natural non-human hosts is important. Geographic Information System and ground verification are important to better understand transmission patterns and predictions, and to understand geo-spatial (micro) determinants of risk.

Disease Burden and Epidemiology

In terms of morbidity, it is important to determine the proportion of specific pathology (e.g., liver disease, anemia, etc.) in a study population that is attributable to schistosomiasis as opposed to other causes (e.g., hepatitis, iron deficiency), to adapt standardized tools for Quality-Adjusted Life Years assessment to schistosomiasis, and to obtain accurate disability weights, including recalibration of Disability-Adjusted Life Years.

Certain schistosome infections have been associated with an increased risk of certain cancers (e.g., *S. haematobium* and bladder cancer) and can have an adverse affect on reproductive health and fertility (male and female). It is important to understand the role of host genetics in these effects, as well as the impact that such genetic effects may have on the ability to vaccinate certain populations. A more advanced understanding of the effects of co-morbidities is important, which may include the impact of 1) interactions between schistosomiasis and other infections (*i.e.*, HIV, malaria, hepatitis B and C, soil-transmitted helminths), 2) interactions that occur with dual schistosome infections *(S. mansoni and S. haematobium)*, and 3) the interactions of schistosomiasis with noninfectious conditions (*e.g.*, malnutrition, alcoholism, autoimmunity).

Host Response, Immunology, and Vaccines

As indicated above, host immune responses play significant roles in both protection and pathology in schistosome infections, and further investigation in these areas is necessary to improve our understanding of these aspects. The discovery and evaluation of potential vaccines is an important priority for these diseases.

Target Identification and Candidate Therapeutics

Treatment regimens should be optimized and tailored towards different transmission conditions. Proteins or pathways that are potential drug target candidates should be identified, and the mechanism of action needs to be defined for both existing and future drugs. Furthermore, it is important to develop and test newly identified drug targets (*e.g.*, orally active ozonides), and to develop standardized assays and/or markers of resistance to praziquantel in order to more effectively monitor the nature and/or spread of drug resistance.

Top Three Research Priorities

The top three priorities for schistosomiasis research are (1) a concerted effort to develop a "molecular tool box" for schistosomes; (2) coordinated field studies of multiple aspects of schistosomiasis in humans (diagnosis, resistance, morbidity, co-morbidity, immunology, genetics of both hosts and parasites); and (3) a focus on drug development, including discovery, defining mechanisms of action, and detecting and monitoring mechanisms of resistance.

In addition to this report, a comprehensive, cohesive agenda was developed as part of a series of meetings and email solicitations involving a broad spectrum of investigators involved in all aspects of schistosomiasis infections from genomics to social sciences. (PLoS Negl Trop Dis. 2007 December; 1(3): e32)

Filarial Worms

Basic Conceptual Research

The conceptual gaps in our knowledge that may benefit from increased research include the following:

1) The interactions among the (recently sequenced) *Brugia malayi* nuclear genome, the *B. malayi* mitochondrial genome, the *Wolbachia* genome, and human host or mosquito vector genomes are poorly understood.

2) What determines the essence of parasitism (*i.e.,* what distinguishes parasitic from free-living nematodes at the genome level), and the immunological and biological mechanisms by which the parasite evades the host are also poorly defined.
3) The molecules that are essential for critical stages of filarial development need to be identified.
4) The genetic basis of infection and disease susceptibility in humans and mosquitoes needs to be elucidated.
5) The role of the *Wolbachia* bacterial endosymbiont in the biology of filariae and ways to exploit this role for disease prevention or treatment should be determined.
6) The increased use of genomic and proteomic data as research tools needs to be implemented.

Basic Translational Research

Areas of translational research that may benefit from further investigation include the following:

1) How chronic filarial infection affects responses to other infections or to vaccines.
2) The mechanisms that determine the interplay between allergy and host responses to filaria (or other helminth) infections, and how treatment affects these altered responses.
3) The key elements of filarial pathogenesis, including the mechanisms of 'homing' to lymphatics, the attractants that direct worms to form nests or nodules and the mechanisms of vascular dilatation.
4) Methods to effectively immunize against filarial infections or against specific parasite stages.
5) Identification of the mechanisms that determine the pathogenesis of lymphatic or onchocercal disease and the clinical expression of these diseases.
6) Identification of filarial secretory products that could be used as leads for drug development for filariasis as well as other, non-parasitic, diseases.

Translational Operational Research

Two critically important priorities for translational operational research are the development of sensitive indicators of drug susceptibility and emerging drug resistance, and new drugs with increased effectiveness against adult-stage parasites.

Operational and Vector Research

There are several research priorities that would effectively support ongoing global programs to eliminate lymphatic filariasis (LF) and to control or eliminate river blindness due to *Onchocerca volvulus* (OV), including overall strategies to protect the effectiveness of drug-based programs. In the area of clinical epidemiology, more sensitive population sampling techniques would aid the detection of infection above threshold levels (below which infection cannot persist) and would enhance surveillance strategies to monitor post-treatment-program populations and potential recurrence of filaria transmission. Diagnostic tests that can specifically determine the absence of filarial transmission or the absence of adult worms in populations are also important as are methods to ensure good clinical and morbidity management. Furthermore, adequate monitoring tools of vector control strategies for both mosquitoes and black flies would be useful, including the means to 1) to monitor black fly infection rates and establish transmission levels, 2) to monitor the development of larvicide resistance in black fly populations, and 3) to determine whether vector control can be a cost-effective adjunct to the current Lymphatic Filariaris or *Onchocerca volvulus* elimination programs based on Mass Drug Administration.

Coordination of Research Efforts

Given the enormous burden of filariasis disease, the extraordinarily cost-effective package of interventions for the helminth NTDs, and the recent global investments in implementing it, it is important to develop global leadership to aid in providing a scientific backstop for this investment to ensure its success. Promotion of a collaborative network of investigators in both endemic and non-endemic countries to address basic research questions and provide tools to facilitate the operational support for the large NTD implementation programs would enhance these efforts. Development of relevant reagent resource centers and appropriate funding opportunities would help in both facilitating and coordinating such international research efforts.

A consensus filariasis research agenda has been developed through a series of meetings and publications including the November 2004 supplement to the *American Journal of Tropical Medicine and Hygiene*.

Hookworm and Soil-Transmitted Nematode

There are numerous challenges facing investigators interested in research on the major soil transmitted nematode (STN) species, which include *Ascaris lumbricoides*, *Trichuris trichiura*, the hookworms (*Ancylostoma duodenale*, *A. ceylanicum*, *Necator americanus*), and *Strongyloides* (*S. stercoralis*, *S. fuelleborni*). Factors that contribute to the persistent research gaps include the following:

1) The pathogenesis of these diseases and mechanism of action of specific virulence factors are poorly defined.
2) It is currently not possible to reliably manipulate STN gene expression.
3) Available animal models are cumbersome and do not always replicate human disease. For some animal hosts, there are few available immunologic reagents.
4) Currently available diagnostics remain labor-intensive and difficult to scale up for population based epidemiologic investigations and control program monitoring.
5) There are limited data correlating laboratory (animal) and field (human) studies.

Basic Science Research Gaps

The pathogenesis of most STN infections has remained poorly elucidated, and the number of specific virulence factors identified for each of the major parasite species is few. Moreover, for those specific genes and gene products thought to be important in infection and/or pathogenesis, it has been difficult to demonstrate a definitive role due to the inability to reliably silence gene expression *in vitro* or *in vivo*. The current status of gene silencing using RNAi in STN species is not yet at a point of broad application, although progress is being made. Moreover, the evidence to date suggests that effective techniques for RNAi mediated silencing may need to be optimized for each gene product, STN species and life cycle stage independently. This will require a substantial amount of research to develop these methods in the coming years.

At present, neutralization through vaccination with recombinant proteins is the most commonly utilized method of targeting or inhibiting specific parasite proteins, but this approach has a number of important limitations for evaluating large numbers of targets. Additional work needs to be focused on developing novel molecular targets for drug and vaccine development using high throughput methods.

The animal models available for the study of STN infections are extremely limited, with few exceptions. Mice and rats are not efficient models for the study of hookworm and *Ascaris*, although they can be manipulated in order to characterize certain aspects of the early infectious process, *e.g.*, skin invasion and tissue migration. In the case of *Trichuris*, although mice are susceptible (to *T. muris*), there are significant strain differences in efficiency of infection, making broad generalizations to human disease difficult. By contrast, the animal models that reliably mimic human disease pathogenesis, *e.g.*, dog/hamster (hookworm), pig (*Ascaris*), and even nonhuman primates, are limited by prohibitive costs and/or a lack of reagents for the sophisticated study of innate and acquired immune responses. As a result, relatively little information exists with regard to host and parasite factors that are necessary and/or sufficient for infection.

The major STN species are also limited in terms of available genome coverage, despite the efforts of the Washington University sequencing project. Clearly more efforts need to be focused on completing the genome coverage of each STN dataset.

Diagnostics

There has been little progress in adapting molecular and high-throughput techniques to the study of STN infections. However, recent progress in the development of PCR based techniques that allow for speciation of hookworm in endemic areas is a potentially important advance. Fecal antigen detection assays have also been developed for hookworm, but to date, have not been validated in large scale field settings. Very little has been done to improve upon fecal microscopy for the other STN species, *i.e. Ascaris*, *Trichuris*, and *Strongyloides*. More effective diagnostics would substantially improve disease monitoring programs, as well as provide for early detection of anthelminthic drug resistance.

Gaps in Epidemiology Research

Due to limitations in animal models for the study of STN infections, it has been difficult to validate observations made in field settings under more controlled laboratory conditions. As a result, much of the work in the field is limited by significant confounding variables, most notably co-infection with multiple STN species and wide variability in host factors (susceptibility, nutrition, etc). In particular, more work is needed on the genetic basis of susceptibility, as well as other behavioral/social factors that might influence infection within populations. Additional information on the population genetics from both the human host and parasite side would be a great advance.

Bacteria

Mycobacterium leprae

Basic Science Research Gaps

It is anticipated that developments in genomics and proteomics may facilitate advances in the development of epidemiological, diagnostic and immunological tools to provide a better understanding of leprosy with the goal of devising new intervention strategies.

Pathogenesis and Clinical Epidemiology

Because there is confusion at the international level about the prevalence and incidence of leprosy disease, a new perspective on epidemiological measurements is needed as well as approaches involving active, rather than passive, case finding. New approaches should determine the true prevalence of leprosy and the actual disease burden. In addition, it is important to develop new molecular tools that could be applied to study transmission.

It is important to develop the means to detect and treat *M. leprae* infection prior to the development of clinical symptoms in order to prevent both nerve function impairment (NFI) and nerve damage.

Diagnostics

Within the realm of diagnostic development, the following areas are important: increased epidemiological studies; studies to assess the effect of interventions; development of methods to detect preclinical and latent infection in order to provide early diagnosis, identify individuals at risk and monitor treatment; and creation of specific diagnostic methods based on cell mediated immunity.

Host Response, Immunology, and Vaccines

New molecular tools could be used to identify *M. leprae*-specific T-cell responses and to predict the risk of disease in affected populations.

As leprosy is also caused by *Mycobacterium*, progress made in tuberculosis vaccines could stimulate leprosy vaccine research. Furthermore, since many people have natural immunity to leprosy, there is potential for immunotherapy in susceptible individuals.

Target Identification and Candidate Therapeutics

It is important to determine the minimum length of effective multi-drug therapy (MDT) and to develop new molecular tools to detect drug resistance and define its extent. Alternatives to standard MDT therapy are important and new antituberculosis therapeutics in development could have a positive impact on the identification of new leprosy therapeutics.

Resources

Cohorts are important for implementation and testing of potential interventions, including MDT, chemoprophylaxis, and immunotherapy, and for understanding, treating and preventing NFI and leprosy reactions. The assembly of such cohorts requires investment, training, collaboration within and outside the leprosy research community (*e.g.,* TB research community, disability services), cooperation with government health services and with International Federation of Anti-Leprosy Associations (ILEP) and other non-governmental organizations (NGOs), support for established consortia (*e.g.,* Initiative for Diagnostic and Epidemiological Assays for Leprosy (IDEAL)), and maintenance of "core" labs and facilities (*e.g.*, leprosy endemic sites and personnel and resource centers (see above)). Further, the maintenance of laboratories in leprosy endemic sites and multidisciplinary research consortia are important.

Collaborative Needs

The continued collaboration between clinical sites and research laboratories is important. Multidisciplinary approaches may help to address key areas in leprosy research. In addition to collaborative funding efforts, advocacy will be important for sustaining and expanding research and program efforts in leprosy.

Mycobacterium Ulcerans

Research Gaps

The ecology of *M. ulcerans* is unclear. It is not known where in the environment it is amplified or how transmission occurs. It is also not clear if there are anthropogenic environmental changes that are responsible for the recent spread and increase in disease. In terms of pathogenesis, it is not clear under what conditions production of the toxin mycolactone is favored or the role of the extracellular matrix in pathogenesis.

Diagnostics

The development of a simple, rapid diagnostic field test for Buruli Ulcer is an important priority.

Therapeutics

It is important to optimize antibiotic therapy and to determine if an antibiotic regimen can cure small Buruli ulcer lesions before they progress to larger lesions requiring surgical intervention.

Chlamydia trachomatis

Basic Science Research Gaps

Advances in trachoma disease prevention and treatment could be facilitated by the following:

1) a system for genetic transformation,
2) an understanding of the molecular and cellular basis for chlamydia immunity,
3) a determination of whether subtle differences between trachoma strains are clinically important,
4) a determination of whether bacterial variants affect transmission, infectious load, clinical severity, or risk of sequelae, and
5) a determination of whether current strain-typing methods are optimal or if there is a need for more informative typing methods.

Diagnostics

The development of point of care diagnostic is needed in order to determine whether individuals need to be retreated with antibiotics.

Pathogenesis Knowledge Gaps

Corneal scarring associated with *C. trachomatis* infection is the proximal cause of blindness in trachoma. However, it is not clear why scarring appears so late in the disease process and why scarring only develops in some individuals. It is also not clear if host genetics or specific host responses are involved in this process. A possibility for studying this issue would be developing and/or expanding the non-human primate model for pathogenesis and immunity.

Vaccines

It is not evident if a vaccine is still the best approach for true eradication of trachoma, but if so, it is important to identify pathway(s) that are suitable for vaccine development.

Opportunities from the SAFE Intervention

There is an opportunity to gain information about a number of aspects of trachoma disease and public health intervention from the SAFE Program. SAFE is a WHO initiative designed to reduce blindness that is associated with long-term infections with *C. trachomatis*. The intervention consists of four aspects: **S**urgery, **A**ntibiotics, **F**ace washing and **E**nvironmental change. The surgical component is a simple procedure that a health-care worker can be trained to do. The antibiotic component consists of a single dose of azithromycin, which Pfizer is committed to providing for every infected person in the world. There are a number of research and practical questions that remain to be answered. It is not clear if the surgical techniques can be improved effectively. With respect to the antibiotic regimen, the questions include: what percent population coverage is required for the intervention to be successful; what is the appropriate time interval to re-treatment (6 months versus 12 months); what is the appropriate age at which children should begin treatment (less than 6 months or less than 12 months); when should treatment of a community stop; and can mass antimicrobial treatment eliminate trachoma at the community level over the long term.

With respect to the face washing and environmental aspects of the SAFE intervention, there are considerable problems with both the indicators and the effectiveness of these interventions. Thus, it is not clear to what extent an 'unclean face' is a cause versus an effect of trachoma transmission, nor is it clear how programs should prioritize the face washing and environmental aspects. Similarly, it is unclear as to whether epidemiological, risk, or disease features are the most important predictor of successful interventions in given communities, or if all three contribute and have an interactive effect.

Natural History, Mathematical Modeling

An issue related to the SAFE intervention is how mathematical modeling could facilitate intervention approaches. Too often mathematical transmission models in the literature are not tied with existing data and are not validated.

Community-wide treatments for trachoma offer a unique situation to study such models as there is specificity in the time of treatment, the persons treated and the ability to determine infection status. Thus, it is possible that trachoma elimination programs could provide data for infectious disease models and could answer the question as to whether antibiotics can eradicate an infectious disease.

Intervention Programs

A potential beneficial effect of integrated NTD programs could be that mass azithromycin treatments may reduce respiratory, diarrheal and skin diseases. Cost-effectiveness could be achieved by coordinating the trachoma programs with other NTD intervention programs.

In: Neglected Tropical Diseases
Editor: Ronald J. Davidson
ISBN: 978-1-61324-387-9

Chapter 3

WASH AWAY NTDS: PREVENTING NEGLECTED TROPICAL DISEASES (NTDS) AND OTHER ILLNESSES WITH WATER, SANITATION, & HYGIENE (WASH) INTERVENTIONS*

Department of Health and Human Services

WHAT ARE THE PROBLEMS?

At present, 884 million people do not have access to improved water sources and 2.6 billion people lack access to improved sanitation.[1] At any given time, close to half the people living in the developing world are suffering from one or more diseases associated with inadequate water, sanitation, and hygiene (WASH).[2] The most recognized WASH disease is diarrheal illness, which causes more than 1.5 million deaths worldwide every year, mostly among children younger than five years of age.[3] Millions more suffer from devastating WASH-related neglected tropical diseases (NTDs), such as soil-transmitted helminthiases (STHs), Guinea worm disease (GWD), trachoma, and schistosomiasis.

---

* This is an edited, reformatted and augmented version of a Department of Health and Human Services publication.

WHAT IS THE IMPACT?

Improved WASH is a critical element in preventing disease in the world's poorest countries. This involves improving access to safe water, managing human excreta, improving hygiene, and enhancing targeted environmental management. Such improvements can lead to improved health, poverty reduction, and socio-economic development. For example:

- More than 1 billion people are infected with STHs, some of whom suffer learning impairment, massive diarrhea, or anemia.[4] STHs are associated with at least 12,000 deaths each year.[5] Improved WASH can result in a 29% median reduction in illness from *Ascaris*, one of the STH worms.[6]
- GWD is one of the few infectious diseases solely spread by contaminated water. It causes prolonged disability that negatively impacts agricultural and animal husbandry activities. GWD causes millions of dollars in economic losses each year and decreases school attendance by 60% in some highly endemic villages.[7,8,9] Improved water supplies can result in a 78% median reduction in GWD.[6]
- Trachoma is the leading cause of preventable blindness with approximately 8 million people worldwide blind and an estimated 84 million people in need of treatment.[10] The spread of trachoma is strongly related to overcrowding, the lack of water for washing the face and hands, and inadequate disposal of human and animal waste.[11] Improving WASH can reduce trachoma by 27%.[6]
- About 200 million people are infected with schistosomiasis,[12] which causes tens of thousands of deaths every year, mostly in Sub-Saharan Africa.[5] Schistosomiasis results from the unsanitary disposal of human waste and the absence of nearby sources of safe water. Basic sanitation can reduce this disease by up to 77%.[6]

WHAT CAN PROGRAMS DO?

Integration

Current programs to address STH, trachoma, and schistosomiasis focus mostly on mass drug administration (MDA).[13] These drug-based control programs have expanded dramatically over the past decade and are now reaching hundreds of millions of people each year. [14,15]

However, with limited public health resources, the long-term sustainability of such treatment programs would be improved by placing a greater emphasis on prevention in addition to MDAs.

Sustainability

The integration of WASH interventions into NTD programs is just the first step. WASH infrastructure is already available in some areas where NTDs are common. However, such infrastructure is often not sustainable because of inadequate maintenance, insufficient training for repairs, and inadequate financial resources for operation. Why is this important?

- In Ethiopia, a survey found that 29% of hand pumps and 33% of mechanized boreholes in rural areas were not working because of maintenance problems.[2]
- In Rwanda, an estimated one-third of rural water infrastructure requires rehabilitation.[2]

WASH interventions can provide the needed disease-prevention components for NTD and other water-related health programs only if such interventions are sustainably integrated.

What Is CDC Doing to Address These Problems?

CDC is uniquely positioned to make a positive health impact by helping countries integrate WASH interventions into existing NTD programs. CDC's support to countries builds on the agency's core competencies of surveillance, operational research, translation of research to practice, and monitoring and evaluation. This effort requires evaluation of the effectiveness, cost, accessibility, and sustainability of different interventions. CDC's WASH Away NTDs Program is leveraging the agency's strong relationships with other international health organizations, academic institutions, non-governmental organizations, and foreign ministries of health to:

- Evaluate the effectiveness and impact of a comprehensive WASH package on WASH-related diseases.
- Study the enabling factors and barriers to WASH delivery and integration within NTD and diarrheal disease programs.
- Assess the cost and sustainability of integrated WASH interventions.

Findings from these evaluations can be used to develop evidence-based recommendations to successfully and sustainability integrate WASH into existing NTD programs.

04/2010

REFERENCES

[1] WHO/UNICEF Joint Monitoring Programme for Water Supply and Sanitation (JMP). Progress on Sanitation and Drinking-Water. World Health Organization and UNICEF, 2010. Available at: http:// whqlibdoc.who.int/publications/2010/9789241563956 eng full text.pdf.

[2] UNDP. Human Development Report 2006. Beyond scarcity: power, poverty and the global water crisis. Available at: http://hdr.undp.org/en/ reports/global/hdr2006/.

[3] World Health Organization and United Nations Children's Fund Joint Monitoring Programme for Water Supply and Sanitation (JMP). Progress on Drinking Water and Sanitation: Special Focus on Sanitation. UNICEF, New York and WHO, Geneva, 2008. Available at:

[4] http://www.who.int/water sanitation health/monitoring/jmp2008/ en/index. html.

[5] World Health Organization. Soil-transmitted helminthes. Available at: http://www.who.int/intestinal worms/en/index.html.

[6] World Health Organization. The World Health Report 2002. Available at http://www.who.int/whr/2002/en/index.html.

[7] Esry SA, et al. 1991. Effects of Improved Water Supply and Sanitation on Ascaris, Diarrhea, Dracunculiasis, Hookworm Infection, Schistosomiasis, and Trachoma. Bulletin of the World Health Organization 69 (5):609-21.

[8] Hopkins DR, Ruiz-Tiben E, Ruebush TK, et al. Dracunculiasis Eradication: Delayed, Not Denied. Am J Trop Med Hyg. 2000;62 (2):163-8.

[9] Hopkins DR, Hopkins EM. Guinea Worm: The End in Sight. In: Medical and Health Annual, E. Bernstein ed. Encyclopedia Britanica Inc., 1991 Chicago.

[10] Ruiz-Tiben E, Hopkins DR. Dracunculiasis (Guinea worm disease) eradication. Adv Parasitol. 2006;61:275- 309.

[11] World Health Organization. Trachoma. Available at: http://www. who.int/blindness

[12] World Health Organization. Water-related Diseases: Trachoma. Available at: http://www.who.int/water sanitation health/diseases/ trachoma/en/.World Health Organization. Schistosomiasis. Available at: http://www.who.int/schistosomiasis

[13] World Health Organization. Neglected Tropical Diseases: Hidden Successes, Emerging Opportunities. Available at: http://whqlibdoc. who.int/publications/2009/9789241598705 eng.pdf.

[14] All-Parliamentary Group on Malaria and Neglected Tropical Diseases (APPMG). The Neglected Tropical Diseases: A challenge we could rise to—will we? Available at: http://www.who.int/neglected diseases/ diseases/NTD Report APPMG.pdf.

[15] Hotez PJ, Fenwick A, Savioli L, Molyneux DH. Rescuing the bottom billion through control of neglected tropical diseases. Lancet. 2009 May 2; 373(9674):1570-5.

INDEX

C

I

J

K

L

M

N

O

P

T

U